The Complete Guide to

MEDICAID AND NURSING HOME

COSTS

How to Keep Your Family Assets Protected

REVISED 2ND EDITION

Atlantic Publishing Group, Inc.
Foreword by: Brandon Pike, licensed Senior Service
Representative

THE COMPLETE GUIDE TO MEDICAID AND NURSING HOME COSTS: HOW TO KEEP YOUR FAMILY ASSETS PROTECTED (REVISED 2ND EDITION)

1405 SW 6th Avenue • Ocala, Florida 34471 • Phone 800-814-1132 • Fax 352-622-1875
Website: www.atlantic-pub.com • Email: sales@atlantic-pub.com
SAN Number: 268-1250

Library of Congress Cataloging-in-Publication Data

Title: The complete guide to Medicaid and nursing home costs : how to keep your family assets protected / by Atlantic Publishing Group, Inc. ; foreword by Brandon Pike.
Description: Revised 2nd edition. | Ocala, Florida : Atlantic Publishing Group, Inc., [2016] | Includes bibliographical references and index.
Identifiers: LCCN 2016046724| ISBN 9781620230558 (alk. paper) | ISBN 1620230550 (alk. paper) | ISBN 9781620233535 (library binding : alk. paper) | ISBN 9781620230718 (e-ISBN)
Subjects: | MESH: Medicaid—economics | Nursing Homes—economics | Insurance, Long-Term Care—economics | Risk Management—economics | Risk Management—legislation & jurisprudence | Aged | United States | Popular Works
Classification: LCC RA412.4 | NLM W 250 AA1 | DDC 368.4/200973—dc23 LC record available at https://lccn.loc.gov/2016046724

Printed in the United States

PROJECT MANAGER AND EDITOR: Rebekah Sack • rsack@atlantic-pub.com
INTERIOR LAYOUT AND JACKET DESIGN: Nicole Sturk • nicolejonessturk@gmail.com
COVER DESIGN: Jackie Miller • millerjackiej@gmail.com

Reduce. Reuse.
RECYCLE.

A decade ago, Atlantic Publishing signed the Green Press Initiative. These guidelines promote environmentally friendly practices, such as using recycled stock and vegetable-based inks, avoiding waste, choosing energy-efficient resources, and promoting a no-pulping policy. We now use 100-percent recycled stock on all our books. The results: in one year, switching to post-consumer recycled stock saved 24 mature trees, 5,000 gallons of water, the equivalent of the total energy used for one home in a year, and the equivalent of the greenhouse gases from one car driven for a year.

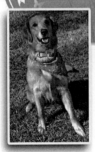 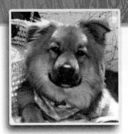 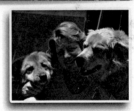

Over the years, we have adopted a number of dogs from rescues and shelters. First there was Bear and after he passed, Ginger and Scout. Now, we have Kira, another rescue. They have brought immense joy and love not just into our lives, but into the lives of all who met them.

We want you to know a portion of the profits of this book will be donated in Bear, Ginger and Scout's memory to local animal shelters, parks, conservation organizations, and other individuals and nonprofit organizations in need of assistance.

– Douglas & Sherri Brown,
President & Vice-President of Atlantic Publishing

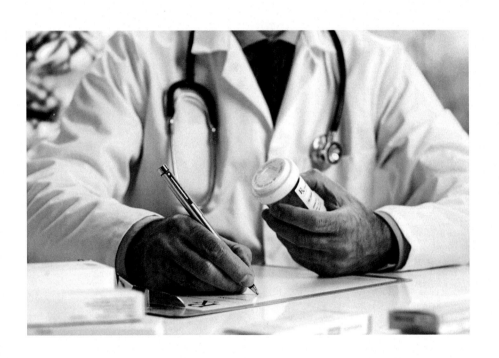

Table of Contents

Foreword 11

Introduction 15

Chapter 1: An Overview of Medicaid.................................. 17

What Is Medicaid? 17

What Is Covered? 20
    Home- and community-based living program *21*
    Medicaid care coordination *24*

How Does Medicaid Work With Medicare? 27

How Do I Apply? 29

Chapter 2: How to Qualify & Sign Up 33

Income..33
    Dealing with excess income...*33*
    Married couples *35*

Assets 36

Estate 37
    Liens on your estate...40
    Medicaid hardship waivers.....................................41

Application Tips..42

Chapter 3: Creative Ways to Qualify.............................. 45

Spend Down 48

Case Study: Julie Northcutt...51

Long-Term Care...52

Gifting 55
    Penalty period and DRA 55
    Value of the gift 57
    Look-back period...58
    Gift splitting...59
    Gift trusts...59
    Long-term life insurance and gifts 60
    Gift taxes 62
    Generation skipping transfer tax 62
    How to transfer gifts...63

Children as Paid Caregivers 65

Warnings...68
    Limited family partnerships....................................71

Chapter 4: Asset Protection Strategies — Safe Investments **73**

Life Insurance 73

Annuities 77

Equity-fixed annuities 78

Fixed annuities 79

Equity-indexed annuities 79

Life annuities 81

Term certain annuities 82

Immediate annuity 82

Private annuity trust 83

Medicaid annuity 83

Trusts 84

Miller trust 87

Revocable living trust 88

Grantor irrevocable trust 89

Special needs trust 90

Testamentary special needs trust 90

Irrevocable life insurance trust 91

Charitable Remainder Trust (CRT) 93

Trusts vs. outright gifts 94

Your trustee 95

CDs 96

Guaranteed Bonds 97

Chapter 5: Asset Protection Strategies — Wills, Deeds, & Your Home **101**

Wills 102

    Oral will...*103*

    Deathbed will...*103*

    Holographic will..*103*

    Self-probating will...*103*

    Living will *103*

    A Health Care Surrogate Designation *106*

Deeds..107

    Survivorship deed *107*

    Joint owners with rights of survivorship.........*107*

    Lady Bird Deed or Enhanced Life Estate Deeds.........*108*

    Beneficiary deeds..*110*

    Other deeds *110*

    Estate recovery trends in individual states *111*

What to Do With Your Home................................115

    Keep it, sell it, or transfer to kids?..................*115*

    Joint ownership...*116*

    Add children's names to the deed *117*

    Transfer to a sibling *118*

    Life estate..*118*

    Transfer to children while keeping life estate...*119*

    Purchase a joint interest in a child's home.......*119*

    Child moves into your home *120*

    Parent moves in to the home *121*

    Taxes on the home..*125*

Chapter 6: Long-Term Care Options 127

Home Care Programs 127

Assisted Living Centers..131

Adult Day Care 136

Adult Day Healthcare Options.......................................139

Taking Care of Your Parents or Elderly Relative...............144

Alternative Healthcare 150

Chapter 7: Single vs. Married — Resources 153

Determining Value of Assets..153

Countable assets...*153*

Excluded assets..*154*

Unavailable assets..*157*

Community Spouse...158

50 & 100 Percent States 159

The Snapshot Rule 159

Purchasing Annuities..160

Chapter 8: Elder Lawyers.......................................163

Case Study: Law Office of William J. Brisk....................166

What Is Certification and Is It Important?.......................167

Preparing to Meet an Elder Lawyer.....................................168

Case Study: The Karp Law Firm 170

Chapter 9: Alzheimer's Disease & Medicaid.................. 173

The Basics 173

Financial Planning..174

Type of Long-Term Care of Alzheimer's Patients 176

**Appendix A: Where to Contact the Agency in
Your State** 179

Appendix B: Medicaid News From State to State 187

Bibliography.. 193

Glossary 195

Index 199

About the Experts 203

Foreword

I would like to shed some light on the invaluable information this book has to offer, which every American can prosper from. Maybe you're a young, concerned family member, or a middle-aged worker inquiring about your steadily approaching retirement. Maybe you're a retiree looking for answers on how to preserve your hard-earned retirement funds while combating inevitable, looming questions like, "What will happen if I get sick and need long-term care," or, "How detrimental will it be to my assets and family." Whatever your situation, this book will enlighten and arm you with the powerful knowledge required to properly and efficiently plan for retirement and all of its complexities. And if you really absorb and digest the wealth of knowledge at your fingertips, you may, like me, have an epiphany and realize a certain irony when the big picture slowly comes into focus.

In regards to my own personal epiphany, the information in this book, coupled with my existing knowledge, joined and revealed every perspective my "realist," level-headed father, who happens to be a baby boomer, was yelling about when he watched his five hours of C-SPAN every night. I'm now realizing, very reluctantly, that he was spot-on and predicted events that would occur 20 years later, including Medicaid spend down. He would gripe for hours about how our government, whether it intended to or not, would systematically wipe out the true middle-class over time. The lower-middle class would be pushed even lower, and the upper-middle class would ascend higher or get forced down to the bottom of the barrel with the majority of the population. The information in this book will expand your horizons and make you think outside the box in one way or another. I know it did for me.

Here, I would like to tackle a little history that touches upon current events within the U.S. economy and U.S. health system as a whole. This will give you an idea of where it all started and some of the many intangibles that have contributed to the squeaky, deficit-producing machine we call a healthcare system. This will possibly (almost certainly) carry on for years to come, potentially drowning many retirees' hopes for a comfortable, stress-free retirement due to health costs, inflation, tax complications and the ever-changing policies related to long-term care. These policies thrive on deception and non-guaranteed values and rates. If you do not plan carefully, there can and will be obstacles that are tough to overcome.

In 1945, on the heels of World War II, President Truman proposed government-funded healthcare, and argued for it from 1946 until 1964, over a decade after he left office. During this time, the baby boom caused a significant spike in the population, accounting for roughly 77 million births from 1946 to 1964. After 20 years of Congress debating what Truman had laid forth, President Lyndon B. Johnson officially signed the Social Security Act in 1965, which created Medicare and Medicaid. Today, in 2016, baby boomers between 52 and 70 are aging into or are already receiving Social Security Benefits (SSB) and Medicare substantially faster than anticipated due to the overutilization of early government- and state-funded benefit programs. Such overused programs include disability benefits and Supplemental Security Income (SSI), which is intended for demographics existing beneath the federal poverty level (FPL), and for those who are disabled. After being on SS disability for two years, you become eligible for Medicare regardless of age, and often, these individuals are already receiving Medicaid or some other form of help.

A number of factors contribute to a national deficit that has negative impacts on retirees: an ever-increasing population that is living longer thanks to modern medicine, overutilization of benefits due to this rise in life expectancy, and benefit programs making healthcare free or very affordable for many. Currently, 40 percent of long-term care beneficiaries are between the ages of 18 and 64, and 70 percent of the population will require some form of long-term care (LTC) after the age of 65. It's pretty scary when you realize the Social Security Trust is on track to be depleted by the year 2034! At that point, the government claims it will start paying benefits from "ongoing tax revenue." The government needs ways to offset the deficit somehow, so aside from just simply raising the general population's taxes, which is inevitable, in 2005 congress passed the Deficit Reduction Act (Medicaid spend-down) to help with the ever-increasing cost of LTC by spending down one's assets and "excess income" just to qualify for government-funded Medicaid.

From this book, you will learn, come to understand, and eventually utilize the best angles and options that will help you maximize asset protection and family legacy while navigating the complex maze called retirement planning. Or, as we in the biz like to say, "preservation time."

Enjoy!

—Brandon Pike

Brandon Pike is a licensed Senior Service Representative in the state of Florida. He currently works for the largest privately owned health, life, and annuity senior-focused insurance agency in America. He specializes in the senior market with health insurance, life insurance, safe investments, and retirement planning.

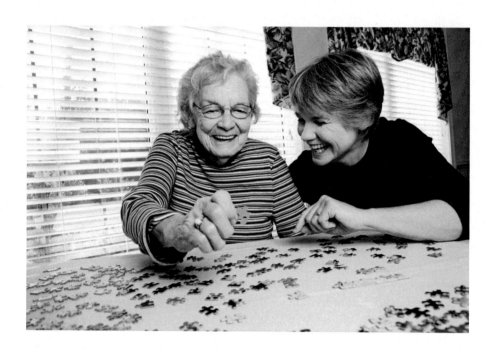

Introduction

The price of nursing home care rises each year. Costs in 2012 ranged from $4,403 per month in Missouri, to $11,771 per month in Connecticut. In Alaska, the cost reached $21,324 a month for a nursing home. All of these costs are expected to soar in the next 25 years. Medicare does not cover long-term nursing home costs, nor does most healthcare insurance. So, if you develop a long-term chronic illness that requires medical insurance, the only program that might pay your expenses is Medicaid. That is, if you qualify with the strict low-income status that most states require.

The cost of long-term medical care can wipe out a family's savings and assets, costing them thousands of dollars. This book is about Medicaid and learning how to plan so you can protect your assets and home. You will learn the latest laws and techniques to help you plan without any previous understanding, as well as reasons it is wise to consult either a reputable elder care attorney or state licensed senior service representative when planning for long-term health problems. These specialists can help plan how to save your assets and eventually qualify for Medicaid. They know the new rules, regulations, and the latest techniques available, and this makes them an invaluable asset as you wade through this tedious process.

All the different laws can make Medicaid confusing and downright frustrating. Each state handles Medicaid differently, so it is important to plan and get professional help. This book will help you understand the issues, and it will prepare you to consult with an elder care attorney, senior service representative, or even deal with the Medicaid agency yourself. The book will tell you about other long-term care programs and services available to the elderly, which vary from state to state, and you will get a good overview of the range of services available.

Take time to plan for your senior years wisely. Consult an elder care lawyer or specialist to help you with Medicaid planning. New laws imply the state can put a lien on your home if you or a family member qualifies for Medicaid, making it even harder to hold on to your money. The state can also file a claim after a Medicaid recipient dies—another reason to consult an expert.

This book will give you helpful information you will need so that when you decide to consult with an elder care attorney or specialist, you will know enough about the subject to make wiser decisions. You will know whether the representative you consult truly knows the subject. Consult someone active in the field who knows the changing laws, someone who works with families and older clients, and someone who has real experience.

Medicaid now offers some home-based programs for the elderly that allow them to continue to live in their own homes, including the Home- and Community-Based Services (HCBS) programs. These are offered in some states as alternatives to long-term care under the Medicaid waiver program for elderly and disabled persons, and are viable options that may be better than pursuing the nursing home route as aging progresses. Improving health and wellness will become a focus as the years pass to save money from incurring financial debt from nursing homes. Many programs are being monitored for cost effectiveness, so this will change some of the rules for Medicaid assets and eligibility.

There is a five-year period after transferring assets that must occur before someone can qualify for Medicaid, called a "look back period." They must not apply until five years from the date. It used to be three years, but it became longer after the Deficit Reduction Act of 2005 was signed. Still, you can learn about the laws and make the best choices by consulting an elder care attorney or specialist who knows how to prepare and advise you on these complicated issues.

Chapter 1

An Overview of Medicaid

What Is Medicaid?

Medicaid is a program operated by the Federal Government and individual states to provide medical coverage for low-income or poor individuals and families. These people commonly have inadequate insurance to cover their needs or no insurance at all. Each state has its own Medicaid office, and different states have varying laws that determine who qualifies. The program has different names in some states, such as Medical Assistance or Med-Cal.

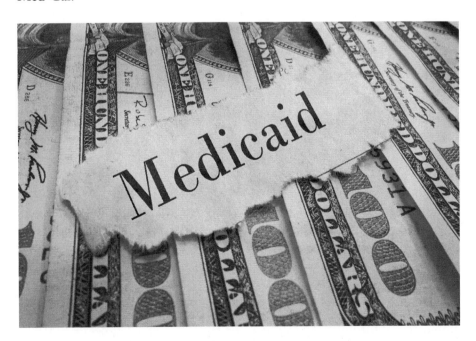

FROM THE EXPERT: *Marty Fogarty*

An issue that Congress has to deal with is the question of what happens when an individual faces a health concern that is beyond their means to pay for. And what they came up with was a thing called Medicare, an insurance program for the elderly. They decided that once an elderly person faces one of these listed ailments, they will qualify for some sort of benefit, payment, or financial assistance for dealing with that situation. That's how Medicare was born, and that's what it did for a long time.

Medicaid is a cousin of Medicare. It's another aid program. Where Medicare is a more straightforward program because we pay into it as we work through our lives, we don't pay into Medicaid directly. We pay into it indirectly through our taxes. When it comes to the elderly, Medicare is financial aid for people with certain acute ailments, and Medicaid is financial aid for persons with certain chronic ailments. Medicare is going to help me if I need a new hip, a new knee, or a new bypass surgery. That's an acute healthcare issue. Medicaid is going to help me when I have Alzheimer's, dementia, or Parkinson's — when I've got a new normal to deal with.

Low-income women, children, and the elderly are some of the groups that fit into the Medicaid program. The blind, the disabled, caretakers, low-income pregnant women, and the elderly who need long-term care or nursing home care often qualify for this program. Anyone who qualifies for Medicaid must meet certain strict requirements.

Medicaid was established in 1965, around the same time that Medicare was created as part of the Social Security Act Amendments. These amendments established Medicare as a health insurance program for the elderly and Medicaid as a health insurance program for the poor. The federal government funds most of Medicaid and often gives more money to poorer states. Average elderly individuals and couples usually do not qualify for this program, as they have a home, reasonable income, and other assets. Yet, Medicaid is one of the only programs that cover nursing homes costs. If you were to become ill and had to go to a nursing home, the cost could wipe out your savings and assets. The average monthly cost of a nursing home per month for one person ranges from $6,757.67 to $9,096.00.

FROM THE EXPERT: *Marty Fogarty*

Look at Medicaid and Medicare as cousins. They are programs that Congress has enacted to help the elderly when facing an elder-health issue. If they have an acute elder health issue, then Medicare is going to be the program that is going to help them. If the elderly person faces a chronic health issue, then Medicaid is going to be the program that is going to help by providing financial aid for a nursing home, or some version of that.

There is a joint program for Medicaid and Medicare called the Program of All-Inclusive Care for the Elderly (PACE), available in some states that chose it as an optional Medicaid benefit. PACE is an optional alternative to nursing home care. To qualify, you must be aged 55 or older, live in the service area, and be certified by the state as eligible for nursing home care. Check with your Medicaid agency to see if there is a PACE program near you. If you cannot qualify for Medicaid and need prescription drug help, you may still qualify for a Low Income Subsidy (LIS), which has a higher income threshold and will drastically help with drug costs.

It is important to know that healthcare information and requirements change often. To see the most up-to-date information at any time, please refer to the official U.S. government Medicare handbook, *Medicare & You*, which covers information on both Medicare and Medicaid and can be found at your local social security office. You can also consult a senior service representative who will help you understand the updates and changes regarding Medicare and Medicaid.

Secondly, for information about Medicaid specifically, please visit **www .medicaid.gov** where you will find information on the most up-to-date federal policy guidelines, CHIP, basic health programs, state resources, the Affordable Care Act, and more. This book aims to provide you with all the information you need to keep costs down and to help you qualify for Medicaid, but please keep in mind that Medicaid specifics are subject to change at any time, so remember to refer to this website when needed.

If at any time you are having trouble finding an answer to a specific question, please refer to **https://questions.medicaid.gov**, which has a list of Frequently Asked Questions (FAQs).

What Is Covered?

Medicaid will pay most medical bills once a person has been approved. Some people are covered by Medicare and Medicaid—this is called dual eligibility or Medi-Medi. This means nursing home stays, prescription drugs, hospital visits, and more are covered. Medical coverage varies from state to state, but most coverage includes inpatient and outpatient hospital services, doctor services, medical and surgical dental services, lab and X-ray, nursing facility services for those 21 or older, and family nurse practitioner services.

Some services are optional, but most states under Medicaid will offer ambulance and home health services to those in nursing homes, prescription drug coverage, eye doctor visits and glasses, prosthetic devices, dental, and in-home assistance.

If you qualify and are living at home, Medicaid will pay for some services. Some states have the HCBS program, and most now can offer this program without applying for a waiver through the federal government. Check with your state to see if it offers this plan and what it will cover. Program coverage includes homemaker and home health aides, personal-care services, adult day health services, rehabilitation for safety and hygiene, housekeeping, and case management.

HCBS may apply to certain services at assisted-living centers. Assisted-living centers must be Medicaid certified to be covered. HCBS will not cover basic room and board, because assisted-living centers are not considered nursing homes.

When a person is qualified, Medicaid will pay full cost of the nursing home bill. This includes room, meals, and all medical services. Some nursing homes do not accept Medicaid programs or payment. If you or a family member moves into a nursing home, find out whether Medicaid is accepted. Nursing homes that do not accept Medicaid payment require the patient to transfer to another facility if money or private pay options run out. It can be awfully upsetting for a patient to have to move suddenly after getting comfortable at a nursing home.

Home- and community-based living program

Changes are underway to reform Medicaid programs for the elderly. Many states offer home- and community-based services as an option for Medicaid recipients. This means they will not be in a nursing home but will be assisted in continuing to live at home alone or with a family member. Because it is so expensive, there is a trend of some states offering options or programs other than nursing home care.

New Jersey signed the Dignity in Choice and Long Term Care Act in 2006 in order to find a better balance between long-term care and community-based services. The state continues to look for models that are cost-effective alternatives to living in a nursing home.

Vermont has developed a program where spouses may be paid to care for family members. There is an option for 24-hour in-home care using a home provider or shared living arrangement. Vermont has monitored the program and continues to look for other cost effective, community-based programs.

In Idaho, a reform initiative seeks to encourage preventative treatment and provide alternative treatment for the elderly. It includes case management, dental, vision, transportation, and extensive mental-health services for individuals with developmental disabilities.

The state of Alabama Departments of Medicaid, Senior Services, and Rehabilitation Services have programs providing a monetary allowance to determine which services an individual needs. The elderly person can choose whom to hire for their care and save money for equipment purchases. Consumers decide who provides care and when it is needed. They develop and follow a spending plan and hire and manage their support staff.

This shift for long-term care to community-based care is the trend. HCBS waivers give states funds for services that do not fit the typical Medicaid long-term programs. Some of these services are for case management, homemakers, personal-attendant care, home health aide services, adult day care services, transportation, home-delivered meals, and respite care.

Texas has the Department of Aging and Disability Services (DADS) to assist individuals who go from nursing homes to community-based programs. This includes some elderly who have behavioral health conditions. For those in nursing homes, the state will build on services that are home and community based.

The state of Washington's Home and Community Services (HCS) provides assistance to older adults who want to move to, or remain in, their own communities by providing personal care services.

A program called Money Follows the Person (MFP) Rebalancing Demonstration Program gives the secretary of U.S. Health and Human Services the right to award competitive grants to increase the use of HCBS services. It supports people who want to move from the nursing home or facilities back into their community. Some states have targeted the aging population.

HCBS services include adult day care, providing services five days a week during normal business hours, including meals and social interaction for seniors and other disabled persons. Some HCBS plans have nurses or social work case managers designed to assist the family or member. They develop long-term care plans and monitor them.

HCBS services are regulated under a Medicaid waiver that allows individual states to pick a wide range of home and community services for the elderly. This program began in 1981 under section 1915(c) of the Social Security Act. HCBS provides these services by waiving certain Medicaid statues and regulations. It allows for elderly persons who are at risk to be placed in long-term care to remain in their homes. This preserves the elderly person's sense of independence and control over their environment. Most states now have some form of this program under Medicaid.

Nutritional services are included under this program, such as home-delivered meals, nutritional counseling, dietetic instruction, and nutritional assessment. The nutritional services help reduce risks in the elderly population by using case management.

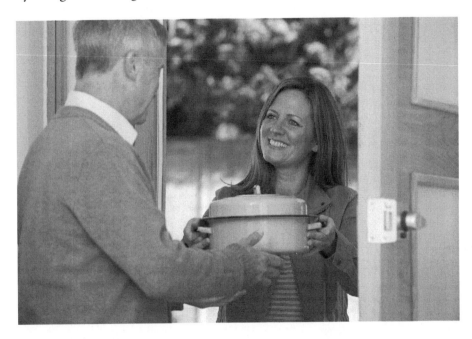

Providers for these programs must meet certain criteria. They must be licensed assisted-living centers, home health agencies, meal delivery services, local health departments, and other such agencies. For nutritional services, they must be licensed nutritionists, dieticians, home health agencies, hospitals, and services approved to participate in Medicaid.

This Medicaid waiver program provides choices for individuals to pick their own provider for the medical services for which they are eligible. This gives elderly people living at home again more control over their lives, which means a better lifestyle for everyone. Choices may be limited depending on the program the state offers. Services from this program assist the elderly who are vulnerable and need more services but do not qualify for a nursing home.

Respite services are available for short periods to give regular caregivers a break or some relief. Many HCBS recipients live with children or are alone and need help to do daily tasks. The Medicaid Adult Day Care program provides services to adults aged 16 and older, including the elderly. It is a structured program that provides health, social, and related support services. It allows those who live in the community to receive care during the day in a social group environment and gives respite to caregivers at home.

More states are incorporating these services to keep the elderly out of nursing homes and help them remain independent and living at home.

Medicaid care coordination

Medicaid care coordination is a service that assesses the needs of a client and coordinates services that meet the client's needs. Some states use this service with Medicaid to streamline care for individual clients and improve its quality.

FROM THE EXPERT: *Marty Fogarty*

What we're taught in this world by society is that you should run out and find a lawyer, you should find a CPA, or you should find a financial adviser. And what happens is you run out, and you go get those guys, and they all help you, and you do your own thing. And then you're going through your life, and you're OK in your 30s, 40s, and 50s, maybe. But at some point you realize, "I'm spread out all over the place."

So, I feel that the name of the game is creating a comprehensive plan that is going to protect your well-being — legally, financially, and personally. And what you need is a coordinated team that's going to be working together to support you.

Arizona has a program for elderly persons who are at risk of having to go into a nursing home. The members can move between the two programs as needed.

California provides the program for those who are seriously ill. The state strives to improve health and decrease the long-term costs of chronic illness by using a holistic approach. California provides disease management, financial and social support, and referrals to improve mobility.

Kentucky uses the the private sector, universities, providers, and others to support the overall care coordination and utilization of supplies and services. The program offers medical services in areas of diabetes, asthma, adult obesity, and heart initiatives.

Some programs provide personal assistance, adult foster care, adaptive aids, medical supplies, respite care, emergency response, and therapies.

Here are some examples of successful case management programs in Minnesota:

- A case manager was helping an elderly woman who lived home. The elderly woman had mental health issues and a severe skin condition that was worsening. She refused to go to her doctor, because she feared leaving the neighborhood, and the doctor was out of the region. The case manager arranged for her to see a doctor in the area. She went to the specialist, and her skin condition improved, allowing her to live at home independently.

- A vulnerable 88-year-old woman was living at home with the help of services and family. She needed several items to remain at home, including a raised toilet seat, a wheelchair, grab bars in the shower, a walker, and a bath transfer bench. The care coordinator was able to get her supplies, helping family caregivers take care of the woman at home. She also bought a blender, as the woman needed pureed food and better nutrition.

- A 74-year-old man had diabetes and heart disease. He had trouble eating right and could not keep himself or his home clean. He was hospitalized several times before he was enrolled in the managed-care program. His coordinator arranged meals on wheels, a home health aide, housekeeping, and skilled nursing. His health and outlook improved, and he has not been hospitalized since he began the program.

- Mrs. J has a history of heart problems and constant fatigue. After Mrs. J underwent triple bypass surgery, the coordinator arranged a temporary nursing home stay for her. Her family was unable to provide her with the care she needed. She did all the paperwork and worked with a nursing home to make sure she was recovering. When she returned home, the coordinator arranged housekeeping services and registered nurse visits for the woman.

How do you know whom to contact to help you with your Medicaid planning?

FROM THE EXPERT: *Michael Guerrero*

There's a realm of possibilities for different advisers. There are the free advisers — friends, family, and social workers — social workers are often very helpful, but there's a limit as to what sort of advice they can give to the public. They cannot, as public servants, provide specialized advice to some people and not others. Family members can be biased.

On the other end of the spectrum, I see a very extensive and professional class of individuals such as attorneys, accountants, and financial planners who have a lot of wisdom around money and making smart decisions. I would say the drawback there is twofold: they're expensive and they're not always the best fit for the job in terms of knowing just the eligibility rules and process.

In the middle of the spectrum are eligibility advisers, like our family business. We are a set of advisers — not attorneys. I have a team of specialists that stay up-to-date on all the complexities of state and federal programs.

How Does Medicaid Work With Medicare?

Medicaid pays Medicare Part B premiums and deductibles if an eligible person does not have second insurance. It is a supplemental insurance for the elderly already on Medicare who need further assistance due to low income. It also covers extended nursing home care. There are also some select plans through private insurers approved by Medicare known as Medicare Advantage or Part C. They provide added benefits for dual eligible individuals. Speak with your local Specialist for information regarding Part C of Medicare and what is known as a Medi-Medi plan, or a Special Needs Plan (SNP) for individuals without Medicaid who have or have had a serious illness such as Diabetes, COPD, Heart Attack, or Stroke. These types of plans have special benefits tailored to each serious illness.

> **FROM THE EXPERT:** *Marty Fogarty*
>
> *Medicaid is a national law just like Medicare. But where Medicare is administered nationally, Medicaid is distributed and administered by individual states. So, what happens in Indiana is different from what happens in Illinois. And what happens in Northern California is different than Southern California, because every state might treat it differently. They might even break it down county by county. So, Medicaid is the same basic, federal law, but it is administered at a very local level, and there are a lot of very different ways for Medicaid to apply. Some places will allow Medicaid for homecare, some will allow it for combined care, and some will only allow it for nursing care.*

Medicare is a federally-funded program providing medical coverage for people 65 and older. It covers the disabled and the elderly. Medicare Part A covers inpatient services such as hospital inpatient care and 100 days of care in a nursing home. It also covers care for terminally ill patients. Individuals who decide to carry only Part A & B and are not on Medicaid or a Part C should be aware of the Part A deductible. The Part A deductible is currently priced at $1,288.00 per benefit period. Each hospital stay begins a new benefit period. If you complete any kind of treatment, including skilled nursing care (rehab), and do not get readmitted for 60 days, you will pay another $1,288.00 upon your next hospital visit, unless it's proven to be related to the same illness. At present, there is no limit to the number of times you may be obligated to pay this deductible.

Medicare pays only limited nursing home care for patients who require limited stay to recuperate from an illness; it does not provide for long-term nursing care. Medicare Part B is optional, but you must elect to decline if you would not like coverage. Otherwise, you will be automatically enrolled. Individuals pay for the plan through deductions from their Social Security check. The 2016 Part B base premium for someone aging in is $121.80, but does not pertain to all. The Part B premium will be higher depending on income. It covers preventive care, tests, screening, physicians' services, and other basic medical services, and has an annual $166.00 deductible unless covered by Medicaid.

Medicaid is not available to everyone 65 or older. It is based on strict income guidelines and need. It works with Medicaid to fill in gaps not covered by Medicare.

The PACE program is modeled after long-term care and acute services developed by Lok Senior Healthcare Services of California. The program was tested in the 1980s and was developed to address needs of long-term care clients, providers, and programs that paid for the services. It allows many participants to remain at home instead of being put in a nursing home or long-term care facility.

The BBA established the PACE program as a permanent part of Medicare and allows states to provide PACE services to Medicaid applicants. The state plan must include PACE as an optional Medicaid benefit before the individual state can participate in programs with PACE providers.

Participants in this program must be 55 years or older, live in the state, and be certified for nursing home care by the state agency. This program became the sole program for Medicare- and Medicaid-eligible enrollees. It provides primarily social and medical services for adult day care centers and in-home services. The providers receive Medicare and Medicaid monthly payments if they qualify. A team assesses the needs of individual participants for services. The average time it takes to process a PACE application is nine months. Some of the services covered are prescriptions drugs, hospice care, and mental health services.

Individuals who are covered by Medicare Part A or B and by part of Medicaid are known as dual eligible. People who have Medicare and limited income may get help from Medicaid for paying out-of-pocket medical expenses or what Medicare does not cover. This dual program is sometimes called the Medicare Savings Program. Services covered by Medicare will be first paid by this program, and the rest will be paid by Medicaid.

How Do I Apply?

You apply for benefits in your state at the agency that manages Medicaid. It varies from state to state, but all states have an agency that administers the program. You can write, call, or go in person to your state department of human or social services or apply online. People on supplemental security income or old age pension automatically receive Medicaid.

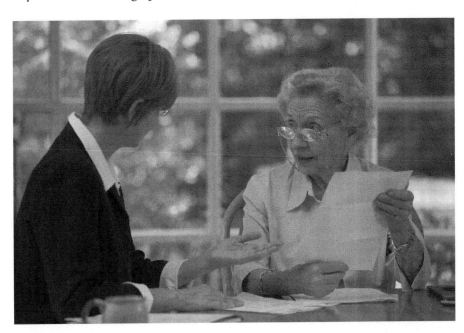

You can find contact information for these agencies in the government-issued blue book or your local phone book. See the appendix for a list of Medicaid agencies by state. Some of the agencies are called by different names, such as the Department of Health and Social Services; Healthcare Cost Containment; Department of Health Services; Healthcare Policy and Financing; Human Services Division; Agency Healthcare Administration; Department of Community Health; Family and Social Service Administration; Department of Health and Hospital; and the Department of Health and Mental Hygiene.

It is important to apply only when you think you or a family member will need Medicaid. When you apply too early, you are often ruled ineligible for Medicaid benefits. You may have to spend your assets or money before you qualify. This can cost you and your family thousands of dollars in medical bills. Often, it is wise to consult an elder-law attorney or specialist who can help you qualify without losing all your assets.

Another mistake some older people make is giving away their money or home too early. Sometimes, this causes tax problems and Medicaid complications that affect eligibility. Gifts can, at times, cause periods of ineligibility for Medicaid benefits.

When someone applies too late, that person may lose the opportunity to have nursing home costs and medical bills paid. This could cost your family or yourself the loss of your assets, home, savings, and other investments. Many individuals have lost all their money to a nursing home and state after becoming chronically ill. Poor planning can mean many months of not being eligible.

When applying for Medicaid, you have to provide income and asset information. You need records of bank accounts, insurances, investments, deeds, and trusts. To avoid delays, collect the necessary information before you apply. You may need information going back five years, so income tax returns are good documents to retain.

When applying for Medicaid, you will need documentation proving you are a U.S. citizen. Acceptable documents are a U.S. passport, valid state driver's license or identification card, birth certificate, school ID card with photo, military card, or a draft record. These documents should be originals or copies certified by the issuing agency.

If you or a relative apply for Medicaid at a nursing home, the nursing home may not expect you to pay until you find out if you qualify. Avoid paying the nursing home during the application process, because it is hard to get a refund. You can appeal a rejection of Medicaid, especially if the person is in a nursing home to stay.

An applicant must meet medical qualifications. A person must prove to be at least 65 years old, blind, or disabled. Disabled is defined as not being able to perform any gainful physical or mental activity due to a physical or mental impairment. Disability can result in death or is expected to last more than 12 months. Often, a trained nurse or worker will come to an applicant's home to determine if they are indeed disabled. The applicant must fail a certain number of tests to be determined qualified. Applicants with too many assets can be denied.

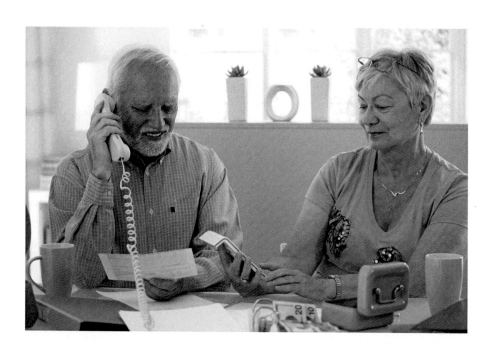

Chapter 2

How to Qualify & Sign Up

Income

The standard has changed to qualify for Medicaid. Before 2012, a single person could not have more than $2,000 of pre-tax income per month, nor income less than $16,000 per year. That figure changed every year to reflect the cost-of-living increase, but lowered in some states after the United States Congress passed the Affordable Care Act in 2010. Signed in 2012, it varies from state to state, with each having a Modified Adjusted Gross Income (MAGI) index, so check with your state Medicaid office to see if your income qualifies. This figure normally includes earned income, such as wages, and unearned income, such as interest and dividends. There are a few ways to proceed if your income is higher than the requirement. Some states offer a Miller trust, a tool that handles excess money for those who do not receive enough monthly income to pay for nursing homes.

The financial eligibility standards change often, so to find out what they are at any time, visit this website: **www.medicaid.gov/medicaid-chip-program -information/by-topics/eligibility/eligibility.html**.

Dealing with excess income

Income-cap states are states that will disqualify you from Medicaid if your income is $1 over the limit. A recent lawsuit resulted in a solution to this problem. States are now allowed to set up a trust that pays the money to the nursing home, and then Medicaid picks up the balance; this is called a qualified-income trust or Miller trust. A Miller trust allows a person medically cleared to enter a nursing home but with too much income for Medicaid to shelter this income into a trust. Still, it is advisable to consult a lawyer to set up such a trust. This trust shelters only your income, not your assets.

FROM THE EXPERT: *Marty Fogarty*

When thinking about doing a will or a trust, most people think, "Oh, a will or a trust, that's just a piece of paper." It's not piece of paper. It's represented by the piece of paper. It might be captured on the piece of paper, but the real work is the relationship and the trust you build up with someone who's going to help you through the transitions that you're going to face. That's the real key.

If you're in your 50s or 60s, it's probably worth shifting your estate planning relationship away from just general estate planner or general practitioner, and get planning done with an elder law attorney. Because you're not planning for next week or next month or next year, you're planning for future decades.

And when you're in your 20s and 30s, those future decades are your 40s, 50s, and 60s, where your biggest threat is that you might die early. So, having a revocable trust, having a basic will trust plan, that's great for those years. But for our 60s, 70s, and 80s, our biggest threat isn't that we're going to pass away, it's that we're going to have a long-term care situation. So, in order to plan for that, you had better have had a conversation with an elder law attorney who specializes in those decades and the challenges that they bring.

This trust allows income to be put into only the trust, not property. Income must be put into the trust during the month it is received and spent no later than the next month. You must put all the income from one source, such as Social Security or pension, into this trust. Sometimes, you pay the nursing home a certain amount equal to the monthly balance, and then Medicaid pays the rest. Income in this trust does not count toward the income cap but does count toward co-payment for services.

For example, Jim has a Social Security income of $1,700 and a pension of $400 per month. His income exceeds the limit of $2,000 by $100. A qualified income trust will be set up to receive the $2,100 that is paid over to the nursing home, and then Medicaid will pay the balance of the bill. The nursing home bill is $4,000 per month, but Jim cannot pay this. The $2,100 will be put into the trust and will be paid to the nursing home. Medicaid will pay the remaining $1,900.

Read more about Miller trusts in Chapter 4.

Another way an applicant can meet the requirements, if they have too much money, is to "spend down" the income. To spend down means to reduce the asset or income to the qualifying level. Medical bills are subtracted from the income to help bring the individual's income in line with Medicaid requirements. Any mental or medical treatment counts toward the spend down with Medicaid. This includes prescription drugs, emergency transportation, doctor visits, eyeglasses, hearing aids, durable medical equipment, psychologists, health insurance premiums, and any expense that meets a medical need. The spend down amount is the share of your income that is over the limit for Medicaid qualification.

Married couples

A married couple has a more complicated set of rules to navigate in order to qualify for Medicaid over someone who is single. That is because each person's income can be treated as separate, and that subsistence-level income is allowed for the person living at home. The person living at home is called the community spouse. This does not affect the partner in the nursing home unless the spouse does not have enough to meet basic needs or has too many assets. The determining income is that of the partner who applies for Medicaid. Spouses are not held responsible for each other's long-term care. Expecting the well spouse to be totally responsible for the spouse in a nursing home would most likely put a dire financial strain on the person's lifestyle. The cost of nursing homes can consume your savings in a few months.

When the person receives $500 from Social Security and $200 from a pension, the income toward the Medicaid limit is determined.

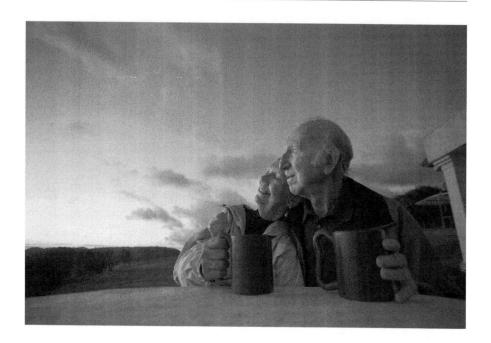

If you own property jointly, any income that is generated will be divided 50/50. This applies to joint bank accounts, payments from a trust, or annuities. If you are living in the community or a house, and your spouse is in a nursing home, you will not have to contribute any of your money to their care under Medicaid rules. The rules vary from state to state about what the community spouse is allowed to keep. Check with your state Medicaid agency.

Assets

One of the most important decisions you will make concerns choosing an executor, or the person in charge of allocating your assets and carrying out your arrangements after death. These can include your funeral arrangement, paying your debts, arranging for the distribution of your assets, and representing your affairs. An executor will collect the assets of the estate, protect the estate property, prepare an inventory of the property, pay valid claims against the estate, represent the estate in claims against others, and distribute the estate property to beneficiaries.

One solution is to appoint a paid executor with no conflicts of interest. This is why some families do not name family members or business partners. We have all, at some point, witnessed or at least heard of very close knit families feud or even get torn apart over inheritance, whether it is from vaguely worded wishes, having an unfit executor or just having several beneficiaries who do not get along. For these reasons, you may want an outside, unbiased executor. The larger the estate, the more potential for conflict, which strengthens the case for an outside executor. There are several good reasons to choose someone other than your spouse. He or she may be grief-stricken or have a serious disability. If you think they may not be up to the job, consider a lawyer.

Most people opt for unpaid executors because of the steep fees that a lawyer charges. Many people choose friends or family members. What should you look for in an executor? A person who is capable of the job. Someone who is persistent, detail-oriented, and level headed, who has exceptional problem solving skills and can deal with medical bills while handling any issues that may arise. It should be someone who has time and patience to deal with paperwork and relatives who may inquire about money.

Estate

Most states have passed a recent law using estate recovery to help with their growing financial burden of long-term healthcare using Medicaid. If you or your spouse is on Medicaid and that person dies, the state can go after assets that were previously excluded. If you own a house, or if it has been passed to others in your family, the state can legally claim some of the assets to pay your Medicaid bill or your spouse's medical bill. This ruling varies from state to state.

Medicaid federal regulations now require this law of all states. There are many circumstances in which states waive the estate recovery law. The law is waived if there is a surviving spouse still living in the house or a spouse dependent on disabled children. If it causes hardship to the family, this regulation may be waived. If the person on Medicaid had a long-term health insurance policy that met with state requirements, this regulation often is used only for partial recovery. Each state will be given the ability to interpret and use this law for estate recovery. It will vary from state to state.

For example, the state recovery unit may learn of the death of a person who was in a nursing home for five years on Medicaid. The person entered the nursing home after March 22, 1991. The state recovery unit will put in a claim against the member's probate estate, especially for unclaimed assets. Perhaps the person had a home that no one lives in; the state will try to get some of the equity from the home. Estate recovery claims in Massachusetts, for example, have increased yearly since 1999. The estate recovery laws have updated the definition of estate to include almost any asset the Medicaid recipient owns. The Fiscal Year 2017 state budget proposal expands MassHealth estate recovery to include non-probate property, allowing the program to recoup its expenditures from probate estates of individuals who received nursing home care or other program benefits for those age 55 or older. This is why it is imperative to work with an elder care attorney who knows the latest laws.

FROM THE EXPERT: *Marty Fogarty*

Congress is drafting these rules. And, over time, the rules have evolved. We can look at the rules as they've evolved over time, and we can see a shifting awareness and a real clarification of the behavior Congress is trying to urge the American public to take. Congress is saying to the American public, "We're going to reward you if you plan. If you do your planning earlier, and if you do your planning more thoroughly with a specialist, then you are going to have more options, and you are going to have better options."

One of the questions they're going to ask you on the Medicaid application is, "What sort of planning have you done?" And if you plan with an elder lawyer — and by elder lawyer, I mean someone who understands how to apply the rules for a client's benefit — then you are going to wind up with a much better outcome in most jurisdictions. With planning, you get to preserve more assets. With planning, you get to honor the people and things that are important in your life. It's less likely you're going to spend down all your assets or go broke or bankrupt if you've done your planning in advance. The laws are written in a way to encourage all of us to do our planning early.

There are always circumstances counted as exceptions to help prevent estate recovery. One such circumstance is if you or the person in your family was under the age of 55, received Medicaid, and did not reside in a nursing home. If the Medicaid recipient is survived by a spouse living in the house, a child under the age of 21, or a dependent who is blind or permanently disabled as defined by Social Security rules, then that person is not subject to estate recovery.

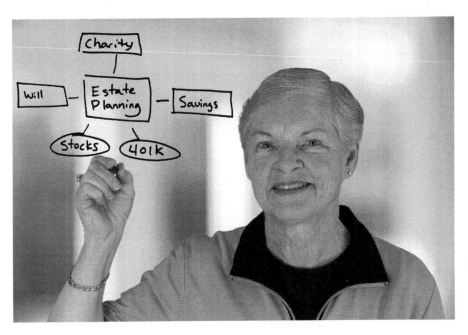

If a sibling, son, or daughter was living in the house one to two years before you entered the nursing home and continued to live there, you likely will not be subject to estate recovery. There are ways to object to estate recovery if it causes family hardship, such as leaving the family with nowhere to live or cutting off funds to meet living expenses.

Most states will file a claim within a year after the Medicaid recipient's death. If the state has a lien against the assets, it may have longer to file a claim on the asset or property. A family may not want to open a probate estate as a means to avoid the state's claim on the estate. Still, some states will file a claim as a creditor to open the probate estate when they find out someone has died who was on Medicaid so they can collect the money the Medicaid recipient owes.

Liens on your estate

A lien is a document filed by a creditor against your property or home that prevents the sale of your home or property without satisfying the debt owed. With the state Medicaid agency, a lien might be placed on the debt you or your family owes for medical coverage and nursing home care. States have the right to collect money you owe for Medicaid recovery. A lien can be placed on a home once a recipient is expected not to return to that home. The lien can be filed if you are receiving nursing home services or HCBS. Liens may be placed against homes or land when you receive Medicaid benefits. Several years ago, Medicaid applicants were not allowed to own any property.

A lien cannot be filed if you have a spouse living in your house, a child who is under 21, a disabled child as defined by Social Security, or a brother or sister who owns part of the house. The exception rule states that at least one to two years before you went into a nursing home, your children, brother, or sister must have lived in the house and remained living there. The lien must be removed if you leave the nursing home and move back home.

The state of Massachusetts uses caseworkers to decide whether to use a living lien when a Medicaid applicant is approved. If someone, such as a relative, is living in the house, a lien by and large will not be put on the property; the property can be transferred without penalty at that time. If no one lives in the house, the caseworker must determine if the recipient will return home. If the recipient does not return home, no lien is put on the property, but the property is counted as an asset toward eligibility. This is waived for nine months, provided the member signs an agreement to sell the property for its fair market value. There are a few ways to release the lien when the property is sold, transferred, or refinanced. Twenty-four states use liens for assets collection and estate recovery for Medicaid applicants using long-term care.

Medicaid hardship waivers

In some circumstances, the state might waive or not seek estate recovery. It might be because the money received would be small in relation to the amount of money used for recovery, or because recovery would cause undue hardship to the family for financial and other reasons.

A married couple should plan for the event that either person might become a survivor when one of them is on Medicaid. When the spouse on Medicaid in a nursing home dies first, the state cannot recover any money if the community spouse still lives in the home and owns the other assets. If the community spouse dies before the spouse in a nursing home, it is not beneficial for the nursing home spouse to get the assets; he or she would then be disqualified from Medicaid. It is important to leave the house to children or other family members.

The state will not claim an estate if it is not cost-effective to do so. For instance, if the value of an estate is $10,000 or less, the cost of selling the property would be equal to or greater than the value of recovery.

If the property or asset is used for a family business, a hardship waiver can be filed. You must prove the property or asset is used for income for family members and that a recovery claim would cause hardship. The asset must be a 50 percent or greater source of family income. An estate recovery claim can be rejected if the claim would force the family below the poverty level.

This relates to estate recovery because more states are going after the property of people on Medicaid than ever before as a way to recover the millions spent on long-term healthcare. Yet, there is a financial exception that allows individuals to get a hardship waiver. This is a way to get the state to lay aside claim on your family estate, especially if you had a family member on Medicaid in a nursing home for several years. The following exceptions are noted:

- A family member is exploited by someone in the family or a
  third party financially without knowledge. For example, the

third party or family member might transfer assets so they or someone else can qualify for Medicaid. If it is confirmed that the person did not know about this, a hardship waiver may be granted if the assets cannot be returned.

- An eligibility worker can prove that denial of benefits will result in a life-threatening situation for the patient. All avenues including transfer penalty must be explored.

- A person might get a waiver if they received assets and cannot be located and cannot return home to have care. Or, if physical harm will come to a patient by returning assets, and that person has no place to return to, a waiver might be granted. If the receiver of the assets will not cooperate and has committed fraud, and the client has no place to return in the community, a waiver might be granted.

- An exception can be made if the power of attorney or person in charge transferred assets but did not act in the person's best interest. The person was deprived of assets by fraud or misinterpretation. Another example is if the person cannot recover the assets due to loss, destruction, or even theft.

- If the person who transferred assets made a reasonable effort to obtain return of assets, a waiver might be granted.

A waiver might be granted if a client cannot access home equity in excess of $500,000 due to lien or legal problems and, if, without these services, the client is in danger.

Application Tips

Applications can be difficult, so here are eight tips to ensure that you get it right the first time.

TIP #1: Provide all the required documents. Failure to do so will delay the application process.

TIP #2: Straighten out your finances before you apply; this allows the state to process the application faster.

TIP #3: Check to see if you live in an income cap state. In some states, a nursing home resident's income must not be above a certain level, but you are allowed to bring down the total number of income or assets by spending down to become eligible. However, some states impose an income cap, which disallows spend down. Checking for income cap will allow you to determine what you need to do in order to become eligible for Medicaid. Learn more about spend down in Chapter 3.

FROM THE EXPERT: *Michael Guerrero*

Don't wait until the last minute. What we hear time and time again is that "This has happened. Now, mom's in the hospital, and we have two days left of Medicare coverage."

TIP #4: If you live in an income cap state, and you have a chronic medical condition that may at some point require significant hospitalization expenses, try to have your assets transferred 60 months in advance of your application. Why? Because that is the "look-back" period for Medicaid eligibility. Look-back periods will be explained in detail in Chapter 3. For annuities and trusts, the look-back period is five years, so to avoid a penalty, make sure these do not fall into that window.

TIP #5: In order to deal with eligibility in an income cap state, set up an Income Trust with your attorney. To learn more about trusts, jump ahead to Chapter 4.

TIP #6: Learn what assets are countable when tallying your assets or getting ready to execute a spend-down. You do not want to decrease your assets if they do not count toward the income cap. For example, your bank account might count, but the value of your home may not.

TIP #7: Check the home equity limit for the year to determine what your home equity needs to be at the time of your application, as these limits are adjusted each year for inflation. If you assume the home equity limit is $500,000, and the limit has been adjusted, then you risk not qualifying for long-term health care costs. Although your home is not counted as an asset, the state will ask you to document the current fair market value by asking for the current tax bill, a real estate appraisal, and copies of your mortgage.

TIP #8: Document your assets year-to-year and make sure your assets stay within the bounds eligibility, as Medicaid will review your eligibility status every year.

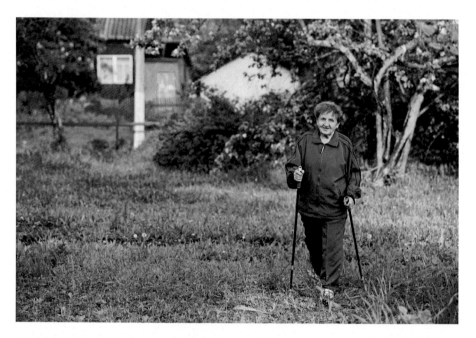

Chapter 3

Creative Ways to Qualify

Do not try to hide your income to qualify for Medicaid. When you apply for Medicaid, not mentioning assets or gifts you made is illegal and will disqualify you from ever receiving assistance. Medicaid fraud carries some severe penalties, and there are several different kinds. Let us review some.

Those who receive Medicaid commit fraud by loaning their Medicaid identification card to another person. Some forge medical prescriptions for drugs. Some use multiple Medicaid ID cards. Some receive duplicate or excessive services for the same health services or resell items provided by Medicaid. Fraud is not limited to just Medicaid recipients, though.

Some providers engage in fraud that delivers the services of healthcare facilities and doctors. They can be dentists, doctors, clinics, nursing homes, or personal assistants who cheat the system. Examples of providers cheating the system could include a home attendant billing her grandmother $20,000 for services she never provided, and Medicaid paying her; a doctor billing for tests never performed; billing private insurance and then Medicaid, getting paid twice; requiring the patient to return for another appointment when it is not necessary; taking unnecessary X-rays and blood work; billing for extra services or for two offices when the patient went to one; and billing for additional people in the family who never went to the doctor's office or clinic. One dentist billed Medicaid thousands of dollars for services she never performed. She was not monitored until a few years later, after which she was arrested and convicted of fraud.

FROM THE EXPERT: *Brandon Pike*

It undoubtedly happens. I have witnessed various forms of medical fraud and possible malpractice on more than one occasion. I have been acquainted with many doctors and administrators in my line of work and have a few I consider friends. I also have written some office group health plans. On more than one occasion, I've listened to doctors, their office administrators, or managers openly discuss and even brag about certain immoral practices. One of the worst I have come across was listening to a conversation between two gentlemen listing and detailing unnecessary procedures, billing and tests performed on clients to figure out who can "burn" through a long-term care policy, and how easy it was to do so, especially with "loopholes."

Another case of fraud occurred with an overweight woman who received a prescription drug for AIDS, a disease she claimed to have. The drug cost $6,400 per month. The woman used the drug for as a steroid to bulk up and body build. It was a synthetic hormone called Serotism, somewhat like a black market drug. The woman stole another person's card, which is considered Medicaid fraud. In a similar case in New York, physicians under Medicaid wrote many prescriptions for this drug, which was being used illegally for bodybuilders and athletes wanting to improve muscle mass.

Some other common fraud scenarios are: a physician bills Medicaid for doctor visits when vacationing, a nurse submits false time sheet for patients who were never there, and a clinic invoices for phantom therapy sessions that never took place.

In one instance of Medicaid fraud, a pharmaceutical company overpriced a prescription drug, thus collecting more money than the drug was worth. As a penalty for this crime, the company had to pay back $1.4 million for three prescription drugs overcharged to consumers. They were supposed to report prices accurately, but instead they inflated them to make money. Two of the drugs were to prevent vomiting and the other was an antibiotic.

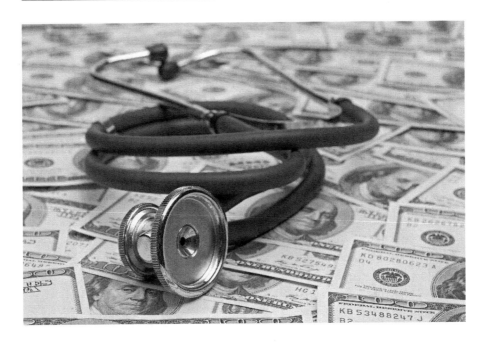

Another company in Missouri billed Medicaid for home dialysis services but overcharged for the services and collected more than allowed. Dialysis removes toxins from the blood when patient's kidneys cannot do it. Some forms of dialysis can be done at home. This company billed for tests not needed and paid kickbacks to physicians. They were fined heavily for fraud.

Other cases include a dentist who claimed to see 991 patients a day and a school district assigning dozens of students to Medicaid speech therapy.

Damages for Medicaid fraud are liable to the federal government for payment from two to three times the amount of benefits received wrongfully. You can pay from $5,000 to $10,000 for each false medical claim file. You can receive a criminal penalty up to one year in prison and a $10,000 fine and not be eligible to receive Medicaid for one year. Anyone who files a lawsuit against you for the government is rewarded 15 to 30 percent of the penalties. In some cases, you will never be able to receive Medicaid again.

Spend Down

Spend down is the process of reducing your assets to qualify for Medicaid. It is, in essence, spending your money until the asset limit is met.

Some people have too much income to qualify for Medicaid when they need it for long-term medical care; this is called excess income. Some people can qualify if their medical bills are equal to or greater than the excess. The classic way to spend down is to pay nursing home bills with your own money until your reduced savings lets you qualify. Another way is to convert countable assets to non-countable ones by spending money on something that will benefit you and the family. To be eligible for spend down, you must be disabled, blind, or at least 65 years or older by the time you need long-term nursing home care.

Home improvements can help you with spend down, as your home is excluded from being counted as an asset. Since you can leave your house to your family members, any money you use for home improvements is wise. Repair your roof, remodel that outdated kitchen, pave that driveway, put in a new furnace, rewire the electrical system for safety, and build an addition for your mother-in-law. These projects will cost thousands and reduce your Medicaid countable assets. Do you need new appliances or to repair your roof? Anything that adds to your home's value is a way to spend your money wisely. How about new windows and doors to make your home energy efficient? Do you need a new heating system or central air conditioning? Have you thought of trying solar energy?

Do you dream of a bigger home? Sell your older, smaller house and move into a newer one. This is another way to spend down your money. Remember, the equity in your home cannot exceed $500,000. Now you can qualify for tax sheltering every two years. All personal property is excluded, so you can buy clothes, shoes, towels, and appliances, to name a few. Do you dream of the expensive Subzero built-into-the-wall refrigerator or space-age kitchen stove? Do not get carried away with this before you qualify for Medicaid, or you may have to pay it back or have it counted. An automobile is excluded, so why not get a bigger, more expensive one if you can afford it? A newer or larger car with more features is a good way to move that countable income to the non-countable column. Do not buy a sports car, but something that is practical and will help you in the long run; perhaps a van for a larger family, or something where you can store your bike for those long trips to the country.

FROM THE EXPERT: *Michael Guerrero*

Don't sell the house. If there's general advice, don't sell the house before you talk to somebody. It may be the best strategy or the only strategy left, but often, it is not necessary. You can qualify while holding the house and using it as a store of value. There's a reason for this. There are a lot of reasons for this.

If you prepay for those funeral and burial expenses, this is not included or counted. Paying out your own expenses gives you peace of mind and spares your family more grief when the time comes to deal with your or their deaths. When purchasing a prepaid burial plan, it is highly recommended you find one with inflation protection and strong transportation coverage. It varies from company to company. For example, if you pass away out of state and need to come home, many plans only cover a minimal amount of miles, then charge per mile from there, which can create a substantial bill. The average cost of a funeral or burial is $8,500 to $10,000. With that said, paying costs ahead of time is still a good way to spend down your excess funds. Just concentrate on value and ask questions.

Purchasing long-term health insurance for nursing home costs is another viable option that still has its place in the insurance world. However, it is predicted that, by the year 2030, many seniors will not have enough income or assets to pay for even the most basic LTC services unless savings rates are increased along with government aid. Although this can be an extremely useful way to spend income, more and more consumers forego this route, as pure LTC insurance is costly compared to the benefit you receive. Additionally, the premium increases astronomically in such short periods of time. For example, on Nov. 1, 2016 there will be a premium spike of 83 percent for government employees. For these reasons, and because there seem to be an unlimited supply of versatile hybrid policy alternatives available now, it is hard to fathom choosing whatever benefits an LTC policy may provide over all the customizable, flexible, ever-evolving alternative options we now have. One perk is that you can purchase long-term health insurance even if you are in a nursing home, whereas most other policies consider that an instantaneously disqualifying factor. Don't wait until you need insurance to purchase or plan for it, for by that time, you may not be able to qualify.

Another popular way to spend is to get all your dental work done, as Medicaid usually does not cover comprehensive dental work, unless deemed medically necessary. Get those dentures made or bridge work done and pay upfront. Dental work is expensive, as there are no service-pricing regulations, and it pays to have your work done. If you need a hearing aid, get one now, as they are expensive and make a big difference in your experience of the world. Check your eyes and invest in good glasses or contacts.

Buy anything that will make your life more comfortable in the long run. You can begin with a new living room set, or a new mattress for your bad back. Pay to get your house as comfortable as possible for you to live in during your golden years; this is a practical and easy way to spend down your money. Get those needed railings in your bathroom or other rooms. Do you need a ramp or special entrance way? Maybe one of those electric home transportation chair lifts? Make your home as easy to maintain as possible. Fix what you have to, so you are not struggling with the repairs later.

CASE STUDY: JULIE NORTHCUTT

Caregiverlist, Inc.; Founder and CEO
Julie@caregiverlist.com

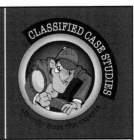

Caregiverlist® (**www.caregiverlist.com**) provides the daily costs of nursing homes nationwide for both private rooms and semi-private rooms. (We maintain the trademark for this "senior care cost list" and call nursing homes in every state annually to update the list.) We also license the information to other websites and economists, such as Harvard University, etc.

The reason we created this cost information is because nursing homes are often an extension of a hospital stay now, and while Medicare will pay for a nursing home, they will only pay for a portion up to 100 days. Seniors rarely plan ahead, and because of this, they need this information quickly when they are experiencing a hospital discharge after a fall, stroke, heart surgery or other major medical event.

Also, if seniors are "spending down" for Medicaid, it is suggested that they first go into a nursing home as private pay and then spend down, as most of the time, these nicer nursing homes will still keep them if they spend down to Medicaid, but would not accept them as a new admission if they are on Medicaid.

CCRC's are an example of a more expensive option requiring a down payment, but will allow a senior to remain at the CCRC if they were to spend down enough so as to be unable to privately pay and then go onto Medicaid. This can happen if they need around-the-clock care and are in the nursing care section of a CCRC.

As an entrepreneur in digital media, Julie Northcutt launched Caregiverlist. com in 2008 to deliver the efficiencies of digital technology to senior care companies, professional senior caregivers, and families. Ms. Northcutt developed the concept for Caregiverlist.com while owning a senior home care agency, Chicagoland Caregivers, which she founded in 2001 and grew into a leading agency in the Chicagoland area, with inclusion on the Inc. 5000's list of fastest growing private companies. She sold the agency to LivHome, Inc. in 2007 in order to focus on developing Caregiverlist.com. Caregiverlist launched the first senior care industry web portal for nursing home costs and ratings.

Long-Term Care

Long-term care insurance is a relatively new type of health insurance that covers long-term illness and nursing home cost. Because of the problems with Medicaid, it is being pushed as an alternative to depending on qualifying for Medicaid. It is actually administered more through adult day care centers, assisted-living centers, home health agencies, and retirement communities. It covers expenses for long-term care related medical bills for the elderly or disabled. This insurance might prevent your family from financial ruin. It also might cover services that help you stay in your home longer. Long-term care is expensive and may not be needed if situations change. There are two types of policies: facility and comprehensive. A more expensive option, facility covers only nursing home care while comprehensive covers both home care and nursing homes.

What is the right time to buy a policy? Some say it is when you are in your 50s or 60s. It can cost between $2,000 to $3,000 per year. Often, the policy covers nursing home care. Be sure you can afford the premiums before you decide to buy a policy, as costs can vary significantly between companies. For example, a 61-year-old female with a preferred rating class, $3000 in monthly benefits, a 3 year benefit period with a 90 day elimination period, 3 percent lifetime inflation protection, and a $108,000 maximum benefit will cost roughly $250 per month.

FROM THE EXPERT: *Marty Fogarty*

It's less about age than it is about the totality of the circumstances. I've had people in their 50s who had diagnoses of Parkinson's or Alzheimer's, and we were doing the planning. I've got people in their 80s who are completely healthy who said, "Yeah, I don't think I need that planning." It's less age-based than it is based on health and family dynamic, or wealth — all those kinds of circumstances.

For most of our lives, we can get by with a will-based plan or revocable living trust-based plan, power of attorney, etc. But at some point, maybe in our 60s, 70s, or 80s, or depending when we get a diagnosis, we're going to note that this is the beginning of a new chapter. And that's when I would start to plan.

Cut the lawn before it needs to be cut. Plan before you need it. Plan when you are in a safe part of your life looking forward into future chapters and saying, "Aha, if I ever wind up here, let me put up protections. I want to make sure there are protections in place there so I never have that worry about the risk of someone taking my home or my assets. Let me do some planning now."

Consider whether the policy pays for just nursing home care or care for services at your home while still living independently. Some policies cover a mixture of care options, so shop wisely. Some will pay a family member or friend to care for you at home. You can purchase a policy from two to six years. There may be a waiting period with out-of-pocket expenses in which you must wait for on average 100 days before coverage begins; you will need to pay your bills until then. A non-forfeiture will continue to pay for your care even if you stop making payments.

Some important questions to consider are the following:

- Will you receive benefits without hospitalization?

- Will the policy be renewed as long as you pay the premiums?

- Does it have one deductible for the life of the policy?

- Does it avoid pre-existing conditions should you disclose them?

- Does it offer inflation protection and allow you to lower your premium payment if you need to?

- Does it include coverage for dementia?

- Does it include at least one year nursing care and home healthcare?

- Does it allow you to cancel the policy after 30 days if you choose?

Which is better: an individual or group policy? Due to the amount of risk group plans, it is wise to go with an individual plan through an independent broker. An individual plan will involve more underwriting. You will almost certainly get better coverage and the cost will be less. There are three types of long-term care insurance: indemnity is insurance that pays a fixed amount once your claim has been approved; reimbursement pays the actual expenses up to your daily weekly benefit limit; disability pays pre-fixed daily benefits once you meet the policy's form of disability wording. You will get paid whether you are receiving a form of paid care or not.

When reviewing policies, look at the daily benefit, or the amount you receive from the insurance company for your daily care. On average, you can select $400 to $500 daily. Find out what the current daily rate is in your state. What is the benefit period? Two or three years is the average for a policy because that is the length of a typical nursing home stay. It can range from $3,600 on the low end to $10,000 per year for a good policy.

The cons include some especially high premiums you may not be able to afford. You may never need the services, or some of the federal insurances may pay for your care. You may qualify for Medicaid if your assets are low. Other options such as a reverse mortgage or trust might work better than this. Long-term insurance may be limited despite the high cost.

What is the difference between a tax-qualified policy and a non-tax-qualified policy? A tax-qualified policy may offer a tax deduction on your policy or premiums. To qualify for the tax break, you must be certified by a health professional as having a chronic illness for at least 90 days. You must be unable to perform two out of five daily living activities. Cognitive impairment must be severe and require extensive supervision. If you claim this deduction, you must itemize your medical expenses. They are subject to age-related limits.

A non-tax-qualified policy for benefits received after Jan. 1, 1997, will not be taxed and does not require certification over 90 days to access benefits. Those who receive care for fewer than 90 days still get benefit payments. They do not have limits of daily living activities restriction. No portion of the premium is deductible.

Gifting

The rule states that if you make a gift to anyone other than your spouse, you are ineligible for Medicaid for a penalty period. Even if your income is within the range, due to your penalty period, your gift will deny you coverage.

A good time to apply is long before you run out of or need the money. Owners of a home with equity over $500,000 will have to use some of the equity for Medicaid. Some suggest a reverse mortgage or home equity line. Do not transfer your home over to someone without thinking about it. First, you lose control over whether your home can be sold, mortgaged, or used for purposes you may not like. You might have problems with creditors, and an improper transfer may result in Medicaid denial should you apply for funds. Watch the value of your home. If the value exceeds a certain limit, that may disqualify you from Medicaid, unless you sell your home. Anyone loaning money for family business will be penalized and if a loan is not repaid, that person may not be able to get Medicaid.

Penalty period and DRA

Gifts to anyone but your spouse will make you ineligible to collect Medicaid for a certain period of time. The duration of ineligibility depends on the value of your gift and when it was made. Whether you are married or single, this law applies to you. There is no limit on the length of this penalty period.

As mentioned before, the look-back period has been increased from three years to five years. So, when giving away money or property to your family or friends, you may want to plan accordingly. The penalty period is determined by dividing the average cost of a nursing home in your state by amount of the gift you made. Let us say you gave your son $60,000 on January 1, 2008. The average cost of the nursing home is $5,000 per month. Then, you divide $60,000 by the $5,000 to get a good estimate of the penalty period.

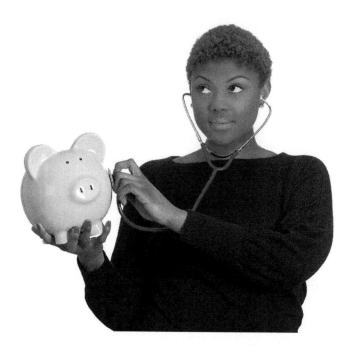

The penalty period often begins when an individual applies for Medicaid and the assets are examined by the state. This new system discourages gift giving by anyone who may need long-term care in the next five years. The exceptions to these rules allowed are: transfer to a spouse or third party for the benefit of the spouse, transfer to the disabled family member for their benefit, and transfer when imposing a penalty on the person or family would put a hardship on the family.

Any gifts given before February 8, 2006 are subject to a three-year look-back period. The new policy of a five-year look-back period with penalties has some of the following stipulations before it expires: the person is in a nursing home or has some Medicaid Waiver services; the person has applied for Medicaid or the person is qualified for Medicaid.

Some states are working on Hardship Rules that will waive some of the penalty period and assets counted. States like North Carolina have lobbied hard to get this into the rules for the state Medicaid applicants. There are many rules to interpret and fight for, but they will continue to work toward helping clients. Elder lawyers are often extremely helpful in getting waivers for clients in Medicaid cases.

Value of the gift

The value of a gift counted for Medicaid is determined by its fair market value at the time that it is counted as an asset. This refers to the retail value or amount of money you would get by selling it to someone privately or in the common public.

For example, where do you find the value of an auto you may want to sell? Using the Kelly Blue Book or getting information from Consumer Reports can determine auto values; remember that one auto is excluded. Bank accounts and CDs are valued by their liquidation worth. With CDs, you only count the amount of interest credited to this account. The cash value of life insurance is counted, so term life insurance has no value. Contact your insurance company for Form 712, which addresses this issue.

You can get an appraisal for real estate including land and homes from a registered real estate agent. Sometimes, a recent tax bill may indicate value of the entire property. Stock values fluctuate every day, so value must be taken on the day you received the gift.

Some people sell real estate or other items to their children for $1 or way below the retail value. This technique does not work, as it will be counted as a partial gift or sale. The amount received will be subtracted from the fair market value. In other words, you sold your second car to your child for $2,000, when the car is truly worth $60,000. The value your child paid will be subtracted from the worth. Then, the $60,000 will be divided by the cost of nursing homes in your state.

Massachusetts has MassHealth, another name for Medicaid, which applies the five-year look-back period for gifts awfully strictly. For example, they monitor your checking and savings accounts for the last five years to see if any gifts were given. All withdrawals will be treated as gifts unless you are able to prove otherwise. A nursing home resident was found ineligible due to two gifts she made to her two sons worth $300. The attorney filed an appeal on this minor gift and the client was excused.

Look-back period

When you or your parent becomes ill, it is too late to transfer their home or money to qualify for Medicaid. For example, if your father becomes ill and enters a nursing home, you cannot give his money away to your family. If both of your parents are living, you can have the home transferred to the parent who is living in the house, and then the state can only put a lien on your home as a worst-case scenario. It will be protected from estate recovery until the community spouse sells it or dies.

Another example: Don adds his adult children to his deed on the house five years before applying for Medicaid. The house is worth $150,000. As long as Don keeps his name on the deed and resides in the house, his share is exempt from being counted by Medicaid. The portion of the house Don transferred to his children may not be exempt from being counted as an asset by Medicaid.

Anyone who wants to qualify for Medicaid should be planning in advance. If you give away assets even five years in advance just to qualify for Medicaid, you can face penalties and a disqualification period under the new laws. Consult a lawyer when planning for Medicaid and give away assets with the thought that you will not need to use this service, as you will work at maintaining your health.

Irrevocable trusts are being used with the new laws so people can remain in their homes. Maintaining and working hard at taking care of your physical and mental health is another option. If clients need long-term care, the children can get money from a trust and sell the family home to raise money for nursing home care. If a person does not need long-term care until after five years, the person is protected and assets remain intact.

For those who need immediate care, a caregiver agreement is an option. This is where children are paid by their parents to help them through a written agreement. The payments made to the children help to spend down the family assets so they may qualify for Medicaid. This child, who may have to take a leave from a job to care for the parent, is paid. This money is considered wages rather than gifts so it avoids an asset transfer penalty. The family member must receive competitive wages and pay taxes on the money earned for caregiving services to their parents.

Gift splitting

If you are married and not a non-resident alien, you can file an election on your gift tax return that allows both you and your spouse to treat the gifts you made as equal. It gives you both credit equally for giving gifts, which is called gift splitting. For example, if you gave your sister $24,000 and your wife did not, you can elect gift splitting so that the $12,000 exclusion is covered by both of you. That means $12,000 was given from you and $12,000 from your spouse. There will be no gift tax.

In another example, you gave the Heart Association $12,000. If you split the gift, it will be below the allowable limit so you do not need to pay taxes on it. This is a qualified charity, so you may get an income tax deduction for this gift. You need to file this when you make a gift that exceeds $12,000. These rules do not apply to Medicaid.

The 50/50 split transfer offers one way for a person to shorten the penalty period for gift giving or assets. The person gives half during the look-back period and keeps the other half. Thus, the penalty period will be halved when he seeks aid. This technique applies to the look-back period of three years, although it is now five years.

Gift trusts

Transferring money into a trust to benefit a grandchild with the help of an elder attorney is beneficial. You can specify when the principal and income will be available for the grandchild to use. You can even specify how the funds will be spent, thus reducing the size of your estate up to $12,000 in 2008. Although trusts own assets, you can still control them. Income earned by trusts that you deposit will not be taxed to you; trusts pay the taxes. They can be used for the benefit of your grandchildren and can be terminated when you choose.

Trusts may be suitable for those who have surplus capital and are sure they will never need regular withdrawals in the future. Individuals who feel confident they will live another seven years may benefit from the trusts. The amount that is invested is put into a life insurance investment bond that is gifted to a Discounted Gift Trust; it will be exempt for gift tax purposes. The owner will be entitled to regular withdrawals decided at the beginning; it provides lifetime income. Often, payments cease when the owner dies.

Long-term life insurance and gifts

Under new Medicaid laws, the government is encouraging those over 65 to take more responsibility should they need long-term healthcare. Many individuals are encouraged to purchase long-term health insurance to cover costs of nursing home and healthcare. Many seniors will not purchase policies because they are too expensive and risky.

With new laws, those who purchase long-term care insurance during the three-year look-back period will find these policies do not cover the cost of the care they need. In states like New York and Connecticut, where nursing home costs can sometimes exceed $10,000 per month, most average citizens cannot even afford policies that run between $3,000 and $6,000 per year.

Some states are working to address this problem by finding exceptions to the Medicaid rules. Others are working with insurance providers to try to develop a long-term health insurance plan that benefits both consumers and the healthcare industry.

The healthcare industry is offering plans with a shorter benefit period. This cuts the price of the monthly or yearly premium. If you do not think you will develop a long-term illness, it may be pointless to buy a policy with long-term benefits. Married couples may be better off buying a shared policy instead of two separate ones. It is cheaper than buying two policies with lifetime benefits. It is not often the case that both spouses need care at the same time, so this saves money. A family history of long-term illnesses might warrant purchase of a policy. For example, if you are younger, perhaps in your 50s, the premium's cost will be lower than if you wait until you are in your 60s.

Anyone under 65 should consider the possibility of long-term care and the necessity of a long-term care policy. This policy helps pay for services that may not be covered but are exceedingly expensive. These policies can give you control over which long-term care services you receive and where you will receive them. It can help with finding home assistance for bathing, dress, eating, and cleaning. Some policies cover community-care programs like adult day care and assisted living services. Other policies cover visiting nurses and nursing home services.

If you wait until you are 70 or 80, the cost of the policy will be astronomical. Some have restrictions on age and health. The average cost of a policy of someone 65 or older in good health ranges from $2,000 to $3,000 per year. Do not purchase a policy if you cannot afford what you need or have to lower your standard of living. Some points to consider when purchasing a policy are below.

Coverage is important. Some policies only cover nursing home care or in-home care. Some include nursing homes, assisted living centers and adult day care. Look for what you need. Some even pay for family or friends to care for you in your own home.

Benefit periods ranges from two to six years or the rest of your life. If the policy has an elimination or waiting period, you pay out-of-pocket expenses for 0 to 100 days, which lowers the monthly premium considerably. The policy should have inflation protection included. It should not require you to spend time in the hospital before benefits begin. The policy should be renewed as long as you pay the premiums. It should have one deductible and allow you to downgrade coverage if you cannot afford the premiums. It should also include coverage for dementia.

Do not purchase a policy if you cannot afford the premiums or it lacks a homecare coverage clause. If you do not want to go into a nursing home at all, consider other ways to deal with the problem. The return rate for this is 60 to 65 percent.

Gift taxes

The gift tax exclusion of $12,000 per person is not the same as the Medicaid exclusion for gifts. Under federal rules, any gift made to another person over $12,000 means you do not need to file a gift tax exclusion, as long as your gifts do not exceed $12,000 per year.

There are no exclusions for figuring a Medicaid gift. Whether you give away $50,000 to one person or five people, it will be counted the same. They will tally up the amount of gifts within the last five years and add the total. Then, they will divide the average cost of a nursing home in your state to determine when you will be eligible. Exceptions are gifts to a spouse or a trust for a disabled child. If you give a gift to someone for $12,000, then it will be counted as an asset for Medicaid eligibility.

With the look-back period now up to five years, purchasing a policy for five or more years is a smart idea. After that, you can give away assets and apply for Medicaid five years from the date you made the gift. Your insurance policy will be in place in the event that you do not get Medicaid. Determining your gift is easier when you have long-term health insurance in place. So, wait until your long-term policy is in place before you start transferring assets.

Generation skipping transfer tax

This tax is confusing, but the premise is that it is a tax separate from income, estate and gift taxes. It is supposed to trap the transfer of property between successive generations. In other words, it allows transfers of property to spouses and children with taxes going to the grandchildren or those deemed to be two generations descending from the person making the transfers. It is a steep tax, roughly 55 percent of the property value. It dropped steadily from 55 percent to 45 percent from 2007 through 2010. Those who transfer all of their property to their next generation do not have to worry about this tax. No tax is imposed on this level. Every individual has been allowed up to $1.5 million as a generation skipping exemption since 2004. There is no tax for this amount. Many get around this tax by only transferring property to next generation, like parents to sons and daughters. For more information on how this tax may apply to you, consult a qualified financial planner or consultant.

This tax usually applies to a grandchild or great grandchild that received a transfer of money or a trust from family member. The person must be 37 and ½ years younger that the person who gave the gift or trust. The recipient must pay tax on the distribution.

How to transfer gifts

One of the most common methods to spend down your assets is called the half-a-loaf-method. A person gives away half of their countable assets. This results in a penalty period where you cannot qualify for Medicaid. You can use the other half for your living expenses or nursing home costs. Technically, you should run out of money by the end of the penalty period and qualify for Medicaid. As of February 2006, the half-a-loaf method will not work with Medicaid with the five-year look-back period, and new rules state the half will be counted and make the person ineligible for benefits.

One method of transferring gifts is for the Medicaid applicant to give away all of his or her excess assets to someone as a gift. The person then applies for Medicaid and this starts the penalty period running. The friend who receives the gift returns half of the assets back to the person who gave it to them or Medicaid applicant. The person now has money to pay for private care while waiting to qualify for Medicaid. This may reduce the penalty period to half.

One problem with this method is that some states require the gift to be returned completely. These are called all-or-nothing states, and you will not benefit if your state is among them. It is recommended you consult a lawyer who has expertise in elder law and Medicaid for your state before using any specific tactics.

Another method is to lend excess funds to family members. In exchange for the loaned money, have the person sign a Promissory note. They have to agree in writing to pay back the loaned money over a specific time period.

Each payment should be equal and paid to the Medicaid applicant. They will use the money to care for their nursing home expenses. After thinking about this method and deciding on the amount of payments, be sure it is low enough to not interfere with the Medicaid applicant's income limits for qualification. It would not work if it disqualified the applicant from the benefits they are already receiving.

One of the exceptions is to transfer your house to your spouse; this is frequently never counted. The assets of both spouses are sometimes added together when one spouse must apply for Medicaid. If one partner has to apply for Medicaid, it is a good idea to transfer the assets or gift to the community spouse or the one who will remain living in the house.

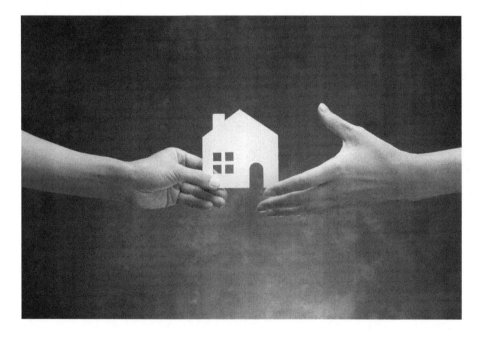

A transfer of assets to a Medicaid applicant's child who is legally blind or disabled as determined by Social Security rules would not result in a penalty by Medicaid. The gift transferred should not interfere with child's benefits. The best way is to transfer this gift into a trust.

A transfer of the home to the Medicaid applicant's child will not cause a penalty, providing the person was living in the house at least two years prior to the parent entering the nursing home. It must be the child's only residence during this time. The child will need to document that the parent needed to move into a nursing home, but because of their care, did not have to; a doctor will have to verify this. If the child lives there less than two years, this exception will not work, especially if the person goes into a nursing home. Nor does it apply if they move out before the person goes to a nursing home

A transfer of the home to a sibling of the Medicaid applicant will not cause a problem, as long as the person lived there for at least one year prior to the date the applicant was admitted to the nursing home. If the brother or sister owns some percentage of or interest in the home at the time, then the balance of home is gifted or given to them.

In some cases, a hardship waiver will excuse gifts made of home or other money if the applicants can prove that not getting Medicaid benefits would be a hardship on their lives.

If you made a gift to your children or grandchildren when you were healthy, it may be excluded if you can prove it was not made to qualify for Medicaid eligibility.

If you made a gift of a luxury car to your grandchild when he graduated from college in 2003, then with the five-year look-back period, it would not be counted. On the other hand, if you make a gift of a car and have sufficient income to cover your long-term healthcare costs in 2008 and then become ill, you should document this. This gift may then be excluded as a countable asset.

Children as Paid Caregivers

It comes as a shock to some families that adult children are not legally obligated to care for their elderly parents. Parents can reduce countable assets by paying their children for non-medical care services. A child can contract with the parent to provide personal care such as transportation, meals, housekeeping and lawn care just like commercial companies.

A contract should follow a few of the following guidelines:

- Prepare a detailed written contract for delivery of services with an hourly rate and time spent.

- Both parents and the person in the service-provider should sign the agreement.

- The signature should be notarized at the time of its signing and dating.

- The rates charged should be comparable to other commercial ventures.

- Find out what other professional agencies charge in your area by calling up a few agencies and getting good estimates.

Keep good records. This is a good way to spend money to get assets reduced for Medicaid.

The adult child who is working for the parent should check with his or her accountant about reporting the contract. Is this is an employee or independent contractor situation? Find out more about income tax withholding, Social Security, Medicare, and reporting to the IRS below.

Sometimes when a child finds out they can charge for taking care of their parents, they say, "I have been taking care of Dad for four years. Can I get paid?" The truth is you cannot get paid unless you had a written contract in place. So, this retroactive argument does not hold any creditability. Medicaid will say you did it out of moral obligation or love, so there is no reimbursement.

For example, in Arizona, a spouse can be paid for basic care of a husband or wife in a long-term care system. A woman caring for her sick husband who gets a disability payment finds this compensation incredibly financially helpful. Medicaid pays for meal preparation, bathing, and household chores. The caregivers must go through formal training and the person cared for must agree to it. Caregivers generally receive about $10 per hour.

Sometimes, family caregiving is not beneficial. According to police reports, an 84-year-old farmer deeded his house to his daughter, son-in-law, and kids. When he complained he was not receiving proper attention, his family became verbally abusive and his son-in-law hit him in the face. The conflict escalated, and the elderly man had to get a restraining order against the daughter's husband, who had moved into a trailer on the property. The daughter also shoved her father into a fence and to the ground. Such situations where elder abuse takes place must be monitored. Caregiving is tremendously stressful and, often, not all families foster caring relationships. It is important to monitor the elderly being cared for at home by a family member, especially when state funds are being used.

Cash and Counseling is a program designed to meet serious problems that Medicaid patients have getting personal assistance in a home for illness. It covers simple services such as bathing, dressing, grooming, and meal preparation. It allows ill people to hire home health aides and have control over services, which gives seniors more independence. Some use his or her own children, since it is a supervised program and is more successful than non-supervised situations. For instance, Brenda Terry gives paid care to her mother, who needs help after a stroke. She is able to stay home with her and be paid by the Cash and Counseling program. Her mother's health has improved considerably.

Louis lives near his parent's house in a separate apartment. He has received personal assistance since 1990 through the Medicaid waiver program. It allows him to hire his own worker. He has a close family friend of 12 years to help him with everything from dressing, undressing, toileting, cooking, and transportation. In June 2006, he switched from the waiver program to a Cash and Counseling program called Personal Choices. This program allows him to pay his longtime worker more per hour than he could before. He is excited about the added flexibility in the budget. He can pay his friend and save money for other things.

Calvin, who is blind, was struck by a car and has impaired coordination. He also needs dialysis for kidney disease three times a week. He has participated in a program called New Jersey Cash and Carry Personal Preference, which has helped alleviate some of his frustration with the programs he used. His sister helps him twice a day and he has ordered a voice-activated microwave with which he can prepare his own meals and computer equipment allowing him to order food online. The program gives him more control and independence.

Overall, patients with the Cash and Counseling program are more satisfied with their care. They receive help with housekeeping, meals, and other household chores. The program relieves the burdens of family caregivers and helps patients with a feeling of independence. A primary caregiver might be the daughter of a vulnerable elderly woman. It gives consumers flexibility without costing Medicaid more

Contracts for paid family caregiving should be made with an attorney so that they meet legal and tax regulations. A contract for services may not disqualify you from Medicaid. It is important to discuss the contract with relatives or siblings to avoid family disagreements.

It is sometimes hard for elderly patients to pay their family members when it is normally something one does for free. Some elderly patients may not want to pay relatives or feel resentful because they have to do so.

A contract should pay the fair market price for services. It should specify how the payment will be rendered in weekly or monthly amounts, or in one lump sum based on the life expectancy of the senior. Some contracts deposit money into an escrow account instead of giving it directly to the person.

Warnings

If you are trying to qualify for Medicaid, it is important to know some areas that could potentially cause you problems. Here are some warnings on things to look out for to make sure you do not land in murky water.

The Medicaid program currently covers about 60 million low-income Americans and 30 million low-income children. This also includes 8 million non-elderly people with disabilities. The raw data shows that 24 states have waivers for non-elderly people with disabilities, and 12 of them have waiting lists. Because some states have a limited number of slots for HCBS, the waiting lists can be as long as 8-10 years. As a result, families are having to admit non-elderly people with disabilities into more costly, unwanted institutional care, or quit their jobs, resulting in lost wages. In most cases, the waiting list is on a first-come, first-served basis, and there is no formal screening to join. Your support service options in the meantime can be found with a home health aide through a state plan, or an in-home health-related care service.

Medicaid pays medical providers through what is called a fee schedule, which outlines the maximum amount of money that Medicaid will reimburse to a physician or other provider for services. The Center for Medicaid and Medicare (at **www.cms.gov**) develops fee schedules for physicians, ambulance service, clinical laboratory services, medical equipment, and supplies. Because Medicaid is a government funded program, Medicaid reimbursement rates for primary care physicians happen to be much lower than Medicare reimbursement rates. Although new health care reform laws have increased reimbursement rates as of late, this applies more to physicians and pediatricians than for specialists, and typically, non-elderly people with disabilities require the care of a specialist. According to Forbes, Medicaid pays nationally about 61 percent of what Medicare pays for outpatient physician services. This, of course, is the median percentage, which means that the low end in some states is lower than that average. Physicians may exclude themselves from participating in the Medicaid payment program, because they tend to wait longer to receive reimbursements from their state Medicaid programs, which in turn increases the complexity of their paperwork and the administrative burden.

The Affordable Care Act attempted to alleviate this issue in 2013 and 2014 by requiring states to reimburse primary health care providers at the same rate as Medicare. Charles Phelps, author of *Health Economics*, notes that following the expiration of the mandatory increase, at least 24 states reverted to their previous primary care payment rates, while 14 are paying higher rates than pre-2013 levels. Since Medicaid is one of the largest items in a state budget, expenses typically soar as more people apply to the program during economic downturns, and Medicaid enrollment has spiked since 2014 as a result of the Affordable Care Act. State resistance is mostly the result of an attempt to control escalating costs. If you apply to Medicaid, your choice of doctors may be more limited based on who accepts what form of payment, so it may be necessary to ask a doctor if they take Medicaid before you apply. Since reimbursement rates vary, the only way to gage your expectation about reimbursements is to find out if your state is paying higher than pre-2013 levels, or if it has diverted away from the Affordable Care Act's requirement.

States have the room to resist the Affordable Care Act due to a 2012 Supreme Court ruling, which gave states the option of deciding whether they wanted to expand income eligibility based on the Medicaid laws introduced by the Affordable Care Act. Because states have the option of determining the degree of expansion, more than 4 million people have no health insurance because they do not make enough to qualify for federal subsidies or state Medicaid programs, nor to buy private coverage on the health law's exchanges. Texas and Florida are two such states which have exercised the option not to expand eligibility.

You should also be aware that some managed care plans under Medicaid tend to have poorer administrative oversight due to recently proposed rules that limit how much these places can spend on administrative costs. A recent report by the inspector general of the Department of Health and Human Services found that half the doctors listed in the directories of these programs were no longer in the network.

Limited family partnerships

A limited family partnership is a legal partnership in which only family members are partners. In one example, parents and children all invest in owning a house. An agreement is drawn up, giving each person a certain percentage of ownership. This is not a good tool for Medicaid, because many states say this is a technique of giving gifts to family members, so it will be counted and not ignored.

The partnership becomes its own entity and has its own tax identification number. It can conduct the same activities as a corporation or individual. One advantage is partners cannot distribute or sell the interest, making the wealth stay in the family. All members of the partnership must agree upon any changes made. It can be settled through arbitration for major conflicts.

The valuation discount is a big plus. A gift at 10 percent in a $1,000,000 limited partnership has lower value than a regular gift given to someone without this partnership. The tax paid would be significantly reduced.

It is useful in reducing gift and estate taxes. Parents can shift wealth to their children through this partnership. Sometimes, children can manage assets for the parents, though they receive most of the income. Upon the parent's death, the assets are distributed without going though probate. The partners cannot make investment decisions, force a partner to buy an interest, or dissolve the partnership. The parents give up assets, but still have control. Sometimes, the parents own 1 percent and the children the rest.

It reduces the value of estate through use of valuation discounts. This means the principal sum of FLP interest is less than value of underlying asset held by partnership. This is due to lack of control and marketability of ownership units. Medicaid may not count as the partnership.

Non-tax advantages include:

- Preserving liquid assets by giving children non-spendable limited partnership rather than securities or cash.

- The children are protected from claims of a divorcing spouse, control remains with the family unit.

- The agreement can be amended at any time.

- You achieve significant gift tax discounts due to lack of marketability

- Control of the partnership, and income can be split among family members based on the percentage of ownership.

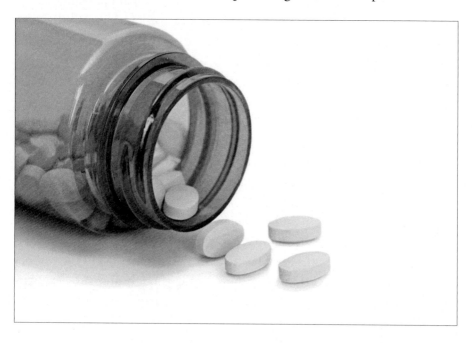

Chapter 4

Asset Protection Strategies — Safe Investments

Asset protection is a type of financial planning intended to protect your assets from creditor claims. Whether you are protecting yourself as an individual or your business, this is a vital step to ensuring financial security. Asset protection essentially limits creditor access to certain valuable assets, but you will have to do so without engaging in illegal practices like asset concealment or fraud.

When it comes to asset protection planning, you should follow a basic set of rules. Do not conceal or hide your assets. Start planning before a claim arises. Never leave asset protection planning until the last minute. Do not legally tie yourself directly to the asset to the point where a creditor can argue that you and the asset are the same. Never overcomplicate your finances. In order to protect your valuable assets, you will need to look into safe investments. This chapter will cover all of your options, including life insurance, annuities, trusts, CDs, and guaranteed bonds.

Life Insurance

If utilized properly, life insurance can be one of the most beneficial tools to combat spend down along with the myriad of options and riders offered with today's policies. There's a plan to conform to anyone's wants and needs. Insurance companies started implementing certain features into policies to specifically cater to LTC. Also, many states now have laws that protect the cash value of life insurance policies. Life insurance in these states is protected by statutes that place limitations on creditor access. Your responsibility will be to research how your state structures life insurance policies in terms of your beneficiaries and the amount of protection against bankruptcy and other financial stresses that leave assets vulnerable to creditor confiscation. Typically, the only way creditors can try to stake claim on life insurance proceeds is when assets from the deceased are in the beneficiary of the life policy's name. The optimal form of asset protection is an asset that is exempt from creditors in an unlimited amount. The reason you should never tie yourself directly to an asset is because this asset protection tool requires you to give up some degree of control over the asset. In other words, both you and the asset should be viewed as two separate entities.

FROM THE EXPERT: *Marty Fogarty*

With regard to long-term care, there's a couple of ways to buy that, but a very popular option now is to buy it so that it's in a long-term care rider on a life insurance policy. So, I know when I pass away, I'm going to get that money. And if I go to long-term care along the way, they can start to get that money and allow me to get a reduced benefit after I pass away, because I was able to use it when I needed it. So, instead of getting $500,000 in death benefit, I get $200,000 because I was able to use the $300,000 to take care of myself during my illness.

Many states under the Federal Bankruptcy exemption laws view life insurance as an exempt property, but again, this depends on which state you live in because, ultimately, the state decides what property you can or cannot keep. Life insurance is among the many personal property exemptions that protect your belongings. Other assets may include:

- Your vehicle

- Jewelry

- Aggregate household value (furniture, appliances, etc.)

- Social security benefits

- Money received from personal injury, worker's compensation, or loss

- Retirement accounts

- Spousal or child support

There are two types of life insurance: term insurance and permanent life insurance. Term life insurance expires at the end of a certain term (generally 10-30 years) and is generally geared towards young families for mortgage protection and income replacement for the family in the result of an insured's death. It generally offers the highest death benefit for the cheapest premiums but does not accumulate cash value and only pays out for death occurring inside the term. However, there are term policies that have an interesting little feature or rider that can be added on called a "return of premium." For a higher premium, if you outlive the term, you can either collect all or some of the premiums back that were paid in during the term, or use the accumulated premium to buy a paid-up permanent policy (recommended). Many companies will not ask health questions known as guaranteed convertibility and insurability. Permanent life insurance does not expire and pays out whenever the insurer dies, as long as the insurer has paid all the premiums. There are quite a few differences between term and permanent policies. The most prominent difference is that one accumulates cash value while the other does not.

The reason for cash value is to create a separate account in the policy that resembles a savings account and serves multiple purposes, which could include supplementing retirement, loans, or withdrawals. The account is determined through premiums, which require a portion of money to be allocated to the cost of the insurance protection. The rest of the money paid in premiums for permanent life insurance will go to commissions, other expenses, and portions that increase the cash value of the investment. If you choose a permanent life insurance policy, you will be asked to choose either a general cash value account (where the insurance carrier credits interest to the account at an adjusted percentage), or an account with variable products (where the policy owner chooses mutual funds to invest the cash value).

Getting life insurance means that an insurance company will often require you to have a medical exam depending on the amount of death benefit applied for and the age of the applicant. This is also called underwriting, which varies between companies. This is another reason why you want to get life insurance in advance of a potential foreseeable medical problem. A normal medical exam may involve:

- A paramedical exam

- An exam by physician

The paramedical exam is usually performed by a nurse or examiner and involves taking blood pressure, body fluid samples, and completing a medical history questionnaire. They are screening for signs of cancer, diabetes, or cardiovascular disease, so you can help your chances by choosing a healthier diet and regular exercise. Avoid the saturated fats and carbohydrates that elevate blood pressure and cholesterol, and replace them with lean proteins, fruits, leafy vegetables and "good fats" like olive oil or avocado. Reduce your sugar intake and drinks that are caffeinated.

If the questionnaire asks whether or not you smoke, admit it, but be advised that they test for a byproduct of nicotine called cotinine. Your best course of action is to quit smoking or reduce your intake so that the level of cotinine tests below the underwriter's required threshold. The exam by the physical is a more thorough exam conducted by a licensed physician and may include x-rays, EKG/ECG, and a cardio test. Do not worry about the cost of the exam. The insurance company pays for it. Some other things you can do before these tests include getting plenty of sleep the day before, limiting extreme exercise to avoid messing with your cholesterol levels, and drinking water, but not to excess. If you do not pass the test on your first try, you can always take it again, but consider working with a life insurance agent who can better coach you through the process. In most scenarios, an applicant will only go through this amount of underwriting if applying for over $50,000 in coverage and/or over the age of 50. Consult a licensed agent on the many types of permanent insurance to find the one that best suits you, whether it be a term, whole life, or universal life policy.

It should be noted that six out of the seven of largest banks in the world have the majority of their Investment portfolios allocated or linked towards universal life in some form.

Annuities

Annuities are considered the cousin to insurance policies and are also produced by insurance companies. Like an insurance policy, you can pay a monthly premium or choose to allocate a lump sum of money. An annuity is a popular type of investment for people to make, because the investment will grow on a tax-deferred basis. The owner of the annuity has the right to change the beneficiary of the annuity. The annuitant is the person on whose life expectancy the payment is based.

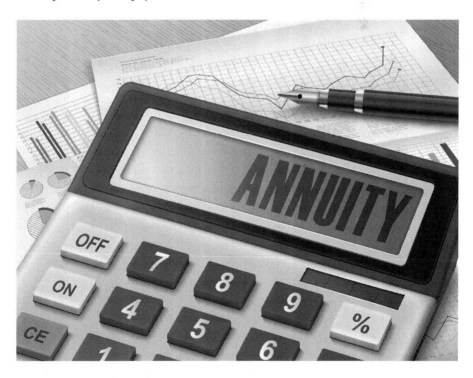

With a Medicaid annuity, the beneficiaries receive payment only if there is a guarantee period specified in the policy and the annuitant dies before the end of his or her life expectancy. The guarantee period is the length of time the payments for the annuity will be made. More often than not, it will terminate with the death of the person. The guarantee period helps if the person who owns the policy dies in two years, and payments will continue if the policy was purchased for longer. For example, if the person purchased a ten-year guarantee period and then died in two years, the payment will continue for eight years. This means beneficiaries of the policy will continue to get payments for eight years, and they would not stop with the annuitant's death. A guarantee period is important with an annuity for Medicaid or other purposes. Take note that many annuities now offer what is called a "guaranteed lifetime income benefit rider (GLIB) that guarantees an annuitants monthly income for life even when account value reaches zero. Most even offer a spousal rider which, if the annuitant passes, it will continue to pay to the surviving spouse.

Another definition of annuity is a savings plan used by individuals for long-term growth and savings. It protects their assets and will be used for retirement. Many use these every year to guarantee asset protection and to have a nest egg to fall back on. It can provide tax-preferred benefits, long-term growth, interest rates, probate protection, and lifetime income. One popular feature of some policies is a premium bonus, where a company will give you a set percentage on your initial investment for allocating your money with them. One very important use for this feature is offsetting losses on the prior investment or making up surrender charges from another policy. Insurance companies provide most annuity products.

Another reason annuities are popular is that they are not taxed immediately. Furthermore, if purchased with "after-tax" dollars, they are only taxed on interest earned. For example, if you decide to cash out a deferred annuity in a lump sum, you only pay taxes on earnings above your initial investment. They also do not drop below the value or price you paid for the annuity. The owner of the annuity has a right to change the beneficiary.

Equity-fixed annuities

Equity-fixed annuities allow individuals to participate in the stock market's ups and downs without losing the principal to expected market changes. It guarantees a minimum interest rate regardless of future performance. It is for active seniors who want to have the comfort of knowing the annuity is stable, but will get a larger return on their payment. It is a middle ground for those willing to take the risk to try something new.

Fixed annuities

A *fixed annuity* is a popular retirement and savings vehicle. It was created for long-term investors who want stability. It lets an insurance company invest your lump sum and gives you a higher return than on a CD product. It provides a tax-deferred benefit that lets you wait to pay taxes in the future. It takes place in two phases: the first is the long-term growth that happens on a tax-deferred basis; the second is where the annuity can be converted into a monthly-fixed income and paid on a regular basis for a set number of years.

Fixed annuities can be purchased from insurance companies or financial institutions for a lump sum. Some annuities are paid periodically while the person is working. The money will earn a fixed rate of return. Often, you can negotiate the price of this product. The amount a product pays out varies, so it helps to shop around before purchasing one.

Equity-indexed annuities

An *equity-indexed annuity* is a type of tax-deferred annuity that exists as a more conservative alternative to the traditional fixed rate annuity. Equity-indexed annuities yield returns based on an equities index such as the Standards and Poor's (S&P) 500 Index, which is an American stock market index. Equity-indexed annuities usually get slightly higher earnings than traditional fixed-rate annuities, with better risk protection.

One of the only negative aspects of equity-indexed annuities is that they are subject to caps and participation rates on interest earned, which limit growth. These are implemented for the company to guarantee your principal. In the same respect, most companies now let you choose to which account you allocate your premium, or they permit you to utilize a combination of accounts.

Companies offer many diverse allocations. The basic options are usually an annual point to point with participation rate and no cap on earnings, which means that a year after the policy is in force, if the market earned, you get a set percentage on the market earnings. Participation rates are also subject to change annually. The annual point to point with cap allows you 100 percent participation in market gains, but caps how much you can earn. A fixed account allows the company to set a guaranteed interest rate for the year. Like previously mentioned, you are allowed to allocate different percentages in different accounts to "diversify" your way of growth.

Before choosing this type of annuity, you need to be sure you will never cancel it, because surrender charges can be costly. Commission fees are common with this annuity, so try to find one that is acceptable for you. Equity-indexed annuities are somewhat complex investments and probably require a professional to guide you. Like touched upon previously, there are three formulas used to calculate the equity index:

- The annual reset formula

- The point-to-point method

- The high-water mark method

The annual reset formula is used during down years in the stock market and examines index gains while ignoring the declines. The point-to-point method calculates the average of the index gains versus its returns, and the high-water mark examines the index value on the anniversary date of your annuity.

Proponents of the equity-indexed annuity point to its rising popularity and respectable gains while detractors highlight the long surrender periods whereby you have no access to your investment, unless you want to take the surrender charge. A surrender period may last 10 years or longer, so if you choose an equity-indexed annuity, it should be with the intention of making a long-term investment. That being said, most contracts allow a 10 percent penalty-free withdrawal each year. Still, they do not allow you to execute a 1035 exchange, which allows you to transfer funds from one annuity to another if you find a better deal, unless you can pass "suitability," which can be difficult, especially in the early years of a policy.

Life annuities

With straight *life annuities*, the simplest form, the insurance component is based primarily on providing income until death. Once the payout period begins, the annuity pays a set amount per period to the person who owns it. It is less expensive than other types of annuities, although they do not offer any money to beneficiaries after the annuitant's death. Those who want to leave something to family should purchase another type.

A substandard health annuity is a straight life annuity that someone with serious health problems can purchase. The annuities are priced with consideration that the person may pass away. The lower the life expectancy, the more expensive the annuity is, because there is a reduced chance for the insurance company to make a return on the money the person invested. The person receives a lower percentage of his or her original investment. The payments are high because of the short-term life expectancy. Other insurance components are commonly not offered with this type of annuity.

Life annuities with a guaranteed term offer more of an insurance component. The person can name a beneficiary for the annuity. If the person passes away before term, the beneficiary will receive the sum of money not paid out. In the event of an early death, they do not sacrifice their policy to the insurance agencies. This annuity comes at a high price.

Another aspect of life annuities with guaranteed terms is that beneficiaries receive one lump sum payment from the insurance companies. This often causes a hike in the person's income, and they have to pay income tax on the sum they receive.

A joint life with last survivor annuity pays continued income to the spouse after the annuitant passes away. The payments are periodic rather than in one lump sum. The cost is higher for this type of annuity.

Term certain annuities

Term certain annuities are a different product. They pay a given amount per period for a certain time no matter what happens to the person over the term. If the person dies before the term, the insurance companies keep the remainder of the value.

This type of annuity does not have an added insurance component. It does not account for health, life expectancy, or the beneficiaries. In the event of bad health or increased medical costs, the price of the annuity will not change to cover this; because of this, these types of annuities are less expensive. The disadvantage to this kind of annuity is that once the term ends, so does the income from the annuity. This type of annuity is sold to those who want an inexpensive annuity to generate some income.

Immediate annuity

An *immediate annuity* lets you convert your savings income to an immediate stream of income for your needs, also called a single premium immediate annuity (SIPA). You will have the security of knowing you will receive money every month even if you live until the age of 110. You can purchase this annuity using funds from your 401(k) or IRA, savings account, life insurance policy, or sale of your home. You get payments regularly either by check or automatic deposit into your checking account. You can choose how to receive payments monthly, quarterly, or yearly. It is used to protect your assets from nursing home costs.

Immediate annuities are popular, because seniors live much longer. Annuities are supposed to provide an immediate regular income for retirement that you will never outlive. They are a contract between you and the insurance company. Annuities are normally purchased with a large lump sum of money by conservative investors. Most are designed to pay expenses over a long period of time.

A 75-year-old male buys a $100,000 annuity policy. Based on the interest rates and life expectancy, he will receive about $750 per month for the rest of his life. If he dies, then his beneficiaries receive the remaining value.

Immediate annuities offer a favorable tax treatment for older people. A large portion of the income is tax-free.

Annuities are used for Medicaid planning purposes, because when you purchase one, you remove the asset from your estate. This is not a good way to remove assets. You should consult an attorney before using this method.

Private annuity trust

A *private annuity trust* is an effective asset-management tool to handle sales of high-priced items, such as real estate, collectibles, stock, and other valuable assets. Many people get this trust to create a retirement plan, defer or eliminate real estate taxes, avoid probate, and protect family assets. It is a product used to create income for seniors. You transfer the asset you would like to sell into this trust, and you are guaranteed a certain amount of payments for a certain period of time for life. The trust can then sell your real estate and use the money to invest in the trust that funds your regular lifetime income. It can protect assets for Medicaid planning.

Medicaid annuity

A *Medicaid annuity* is used to protect your assets immediately from the cost of long-term medical care such as nursing homes. Since Medicaid does not pay nursing home costs if you have too many assets, many people with liquid assets higher than $2,000 are using this technique. A person transfers assets to a third-party insurance company to purchase an annuity that guarantees the owner a fixed monthly income for life.

Some states disapprove of this tactic, but many states have a policy for this procedure. The annuity contract must be irrevocable, non-transferable, and have equal payments over the lifetime of the annuity. Since payments are fixed, you will receive a check for the same amount every month regardless of the performance of the stock market. You cannot withdraw the principal of the annuity once purchased. In some cases, the annuity may be put in the community spouse's name if the other spouse has plans to enter a nursing home.

In the Deficit Reduction Act of 2005, any annuity purchased after 2006 must name the state as a beneficiary in order not to have the annuity counted as an asset when applying for Medicaid. This is the only way to purchase an annuity and not have it counted for Medicaid if you became ill and had to get long-term assistance.

Trusts

A trust is a document with a set of specific instructions to a person called a trustee. It is a legal document enforceable by law. The issues addressed by trusts include: how the person's assets will be used; who gets the assets when the trust ends or the person dies; what debts and taxes can be paid with the trust; who the trustees are; the power the trustees have with the assets; and how the assets can be invested.

Trusts are useful if you are leaving money to people who would spend it before they receive it. A trust protects your beneficiary from other family members who might go after the money or trick others out of the money they deserve. A trust is useful to plan for your own disability or long-term health concerns.

A trust allows a person to manage property or assets for the benefit of another person. Trust property can be many different types of assets, such as cash, stocks, real estate, and CDs. The property in the trust in called principal of the trust. Interest or revenue generated by the trust in called the trust income.

A *revocable trust*, also called a living trust, is one that can be changed by creators at any time. These are not recommended for Medicaid planning. Since the person can change the trust any time, all assets are considered countable toward Medicaid eligibility.

An *irrevocable trust* is a trust that cannot be changed or revoked by the person who creates it. These trusts are more useful for Medicaid planning purposes. If the transfer to the trust is considered a gift, it is no longer a countable asset. Once the Medicaid look-back period or penalty period expires, the trust is ignored. For example, if you transferred all your assets into the right irrevocable trust, waited five years, and then applied for Medicaid, the trust would not be counted. That is an ideal situation that you cannot count on.

> **FROM THE EXPERT:** *Marty Fogarty*
>
> *This is why you need an elder lawyer who knows what he's doing. You have to talk to the lawyer, and you have to say, "Explain to me what the rules are for how an irrevocable trust is going to make a difference for me, versus a revocable trust."*
>
> *The revocable trust will not help you protect any assets or qualify any faster. The irrevocable trust, in many cases and states, will allow you to qualify faster and protect the assets. Congress wrote the rules in a way that said, "If you create an irrevocable asset-protection trust, designed for health care situations, then you can qualify for Medicaid sooner, and you can protect more assets than just the $2,000 spend-down limit or the 109 for the spouse limit." Now, this is a state-by-state interpretation of the Medicaid rules, so every state is going to be different, but that's why you need to talk to an elder law attorney.*

An income-only irrevocable trust is one trust used specifically for Medicaid. Medicaid considers the assets of this trust not countable. The common terms state that the person who makes the trust gives up all rights to principal assets of the trust, but has the right to all income generated by those assets. If, for example, real estate, such as a home and land, is involved in a trust, often the person can live in the house. This trust provides the flexibility to sell assets such as real estate, while protecting principal assets.

Irrevocable trusts give you the flexibility to change your mind. Once the assets are transferred, you cannot get them back. Your use of the trust is restricted forever—you cannot use money for a trip or to pay your nursing home bill. You are guaranteed that your heir will get the asset or property. It will not be sold or claimed by the state to pay for the nursing home bill. A transfer to this deed disqualifies you from Medicaid for five years, so this method should not be used if you expect to enter a claim before that.

Another trust worth discussing is a *self-settled trust*, which is one created for your own benefit. It protects your assets from creditors and others who may try to get the money or property, yet are not entitled to it. Sometimes, these trusts are self-settled spendthrift trusts. In the 1990s, these trusts became popular. Many states do not recognize this trust, but if you are under the age of 65 and are disabled, a trust such as this can be established for you. Medicaid will not count your assets. A parent, grandparent, legal guardian, or court must establish such trusts. You must have a payback clause that states you will repay Medicaid all debts owed through the state. Such trusts can supplement what Medicaid pays for and will leave some assets to family instead of the state.

Pooled trusts under current laws will be counted against those on public assistance, so this type of trust would cut off or disqualify an applicant from Medicaid. It is also a trust set up by a nonprofit organization in a state that holds funds of disabled individuals to be used to supplement their income. In this case, Medicaid would not count the trust. Contributions from each person are counted separately, but all money collected is pooled as one source to be used for the group. If a person is under 65, he or she is not penalized, but some states view trusts as countable for persons over 65. Money can be used for items that Medicaid does not pay for.

Pooled trusts benefit the elderly person who is infirm, some nursing home residents, and recipients of government assistance programs. It can be used for elderly care services, guardian fees, supplemental nursing care, and medical procedures not covered by government care. Other needs, such as clothing, medical insurance, handicapped vans, vacations, and travel expenses are included.

There are three elements to a trust document. The *grantor* is the person with the money who owns the trust. The grantor wants to get assets out of his or her name to prevent lawsuits and for asset protection. The *trustee* is the person who manages the trust. *Beneficiaries* are the family members, friends, associates, or charitable organizations you leave assets or money to.

Before you implement any trust, it is good to know the pros and cons of having one. The advantages of most trusts are asset protection, tax planning, avoiding expense, delay of probate, confidentiality, estate planning, and gaining flexibility.

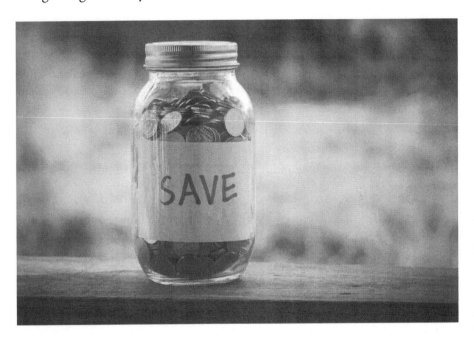

Miller trust

The Miller trust solves one problem — if the person applying has too much income and too many assets for Medicaid — but that is the only problem it solves. Other names for this trust are income-cap or income-assignment trust. The person who creates the trust assigns to it the right to receive Social Security and pension. Thus, the trust is receiving the income, not the person.

If the person is going to receive care at home, they should not give all the income to the Miller trust, but just part of it. For example, if he received $900 from Social Security and $600 from his pension, he should assign only his Social Security to it; whatever it takes to get the income level ready for Medicaid. A power of attorney can create a Miller trust for a disabled person. You would then create a bank account for the trust. The bank account cannot have an opening balance. Then, you write to your Social Security or pension office and have them deposit funds to this trust. It is not a long-range planning tool, but it is for someone who plans to apply for Medicaid in the next few months.

If you have a will and disinherit family members, your will may be an open invitation to lawsuits. If you have a missing heir, that heir may be notified of the pending probate that could result in your estate being tied up for years. A trust avoids probate, and your assets will be distributed to whom you specified by trustee.

Revocable living trust

This is used for married couples in Medicaid planning. It is not particularly helpful to a single person seeking Medicaid assistance. This trust aims to increase the amount the community spouse or person not going into a nursing home is allowed to keep. The property loses its exempt status; this will help the community spouse get half of the assets when counted. You can sometimes spend down the trust by transferring the property out of the trust into the ownership of the community spouse. Overall, if one person owns the trust, then it will be counted by the state for Medicaid purposes.

The revocable trust does not protect your assets from lawsuit, estate taxes, or probate. Because the person who grants the trust is normally the trustee, he still owns money or assets and is subject to claims against it. Its best asset is eliminating probate. It serves as an extension of your will.

Actually, it is a popular alternative to a will as a way to pass property after you die. It is made for management and fair distribution of your property. It can be changed or eliminated at any time, because it is revocable. The trusts are established by written agreement and appointment of a trustee to manage the property. The trust gives detailed instructions that tell how the property will be managed and distributed.

Any competent adult can establish a revocable trust. Husbands and wives often establish a trust together. It can instruct that their community and separate property assets be held in different accounts. A revocable trust avoids probate, because you collect your assets and transfer them to the trustee before you die. It does not avoid estate, income and gift taxes. A federal estate tax return must be filed after you die if your net is worth more than $1.5 million.

Grantor irrevocable trust

A person who could utilize this trust is someone living in an assisted-living center. They need a personal attendant to live in the assisted living center or be in a nursing home. Medicaid does not pay for companion care.

This would be used so the assets are not counted when a person applies for Medicaid. They can make the gift without a trust. There are more risks making an outright gift. This includes the fact that the creditor may attach the gift or seek money from the gift so it benefits neither the giver nor the person receiving it. The child's spouse can make a claim against the gift in a divorce; the person receiving the gift becomes disabled, so it is used for their medical problems. The elderly person can be the trustee to this trust.

This trust addresses these risks. The adult creates the trust and funds it with assets, such as a house, cash, or securities. Money can still be used for the adult, and the person can even be the trustee. It can result in a penalty against anyone applying for Medicaid assistance. If an adult is using cash and securities for income, this money can still be used to assist them.

The grantor is the person with the money or owner of the assets. The trust specifies that this be an adult not entitled to receive the principal distribution from the trust. This means the adult is severing his ties from the assets. The trust also has a spendthrift clause that specifies that the principal is unavailable to the child's creditors. It can hold assets for the child even after the adult dies. It has three elements: grantor, trustee, and beneficiaries. The trustee is the person who is empowered to carry out the terms of the trust agreements. When asset protection is important, the trustee should not be the grantor, too. The beneficiaries are the persons who will benefit from income or assets of the trust.

A transfer of the house or other assets to the grantor can be advantageous. The capital gain taxes can be wiped out on the death of the elderly person who makes the trust. He or she can maintain the trust while making plans to pass them on after his or her death or disability.

Special needs trust

Rules make it more advantageous for persons under 65 to create a special needs trust. They have some exceptions that allow a trust to be established by a parent, grandparent, guardian, or conservator. The beneficiary must be disabled as defined by the Social Security Act. If the beneficiary is receiving Social Security Disability (SSD) or Supplemental Security Income (SSI), the requirement is met. At the death of the beneficiary, the remaining Payback Trust balance must be given to Medicaid.

The establishment of the trust depends on whether the person who needs it has parents or grandparents to make decisions. If not, then a court will have to appoint someone to make decisions for them.

A Medicaid Payback Trust is established to prevent the funds from an estate or personal injury suit from disqualifying an older or younger disabled person from benefits like Social Security and Medicaid. Trust money may be useful for many medical and personal services not covered by Medicaid.

Testamentary special needs trust

This trust is used when a married couple has one person on Medicaid. If the community spouse dies, the assets should not go to the nursing home spouse. This would give the nursing home spouse too many resources and would disqualify them from Medicaid. The attorney would write a will that disinherits the nursing home spouse. In most states, you cannot disinherit a spouse completely.

In Arizona, for example, if a spouse is disinherited, the law says they are entitled to receive allowances and exemptions up to $37,000. If the nursing home spouse does not exercise the right to receive this, the state may disqualify them from Medicaid for 10 months or more; this trust addresses that problem. The community spouse writes a will giving all assets to children except for the $37,000 special needs trust in favor of the nursing home. Because the funds are in a special trust, they do not count against the nursing home spouse. It will not disqualify them from Medicaid and can be used to purchase items that Medicaid does not purchase, such as dental work, furniture, TV, and companion care. This trust can also work for a disabled person without jeopardizing his or her eligibility. A family could set up this trust for a disabled elderly relative, and that would not disqualify them from Medicaid.

This trust is designed to preserve SSI, Medicaid, and other public assistance benefits when unexpected events occur. An adult in a nursing home receives public benefits, and then is awarded an inheritance, or a disabled adult in a stilted nursing facility receives proceeds from a personal injury settlement or suit. This trust will set up the money to be used for other medical and personal care needs not covered by Medicaid or public assistance.

Other supplemental needs not covered are alternative medical therapies, physician specialists not covered by Medicaid, massage sessions, haircut and salon services, over-the-counter medication such as vitamins and herbal supplements, personal assistance, taxi rides, travel expenses to visit family, furniture, clothing, cell phones, vacation trips, attorney fees, and more.

This trust allows a disabled person to maintain eligibility for government benefits such as Medicaid and supplemental security income.

Irrevocable life insurance trust

These trusts hold your life insurance policy, removing it from your estate. Once it is created, it cannot be changed. Once you place the insurance policy in another person's name, you cannot take it back under your own name. You can control who the beneficiaries of your policy will be. You also can define the way they receive benefits.

You can choose who will be your trustee. It is important to get good legal advice to establish this properly, because it will undoubtedly give you tax breaks.

Some people feel these trusts are too complicated and expensive to maintain, and that they are not worth the potential tax savings . You lose the ability to use cash value of the policy should you change your mind and want to cash it in. If your circumstances change, you cannot alter this type of trust.

The premiums are frequently paid by annual gifts made to the trust by the person who established it. The trustee cannot be you, but it might be someone from your bank or an accountant.

You set the terms of the assets distribution in this trust. You can have assets distributed in total to all your beneficiaries immediately, or you can arrange to have certain members receive monthly or periodic distributions from the trust. You can dictate that someone must be at least 25 years of age before they receive any money. You can use this trust to help someone with educational costs or a business start-up. Most people name their children and grandchildren as beneficiaries. A trustee will follow your direction on how to use this trust, pay your insurance premiums, and file it on tax returns.

You can use an individual life insurance policy, or, if your spouse is alive, you can use a survivorship policy. This pays out death benefits after both spouses pass away. You cannot stop your beneficiaries from withdrawing money from the trust, so it is important to have their cooperation for this policy. If you decide you do not want to continue to pay the premiums, you can get rid of this policy is by letting it lapse. However, if it is a whole life policy or a universal life policy, check to see if there is any cash value buildup in the policy before you decide to let it lapse. Have it reviewed by your agent to be sure.

This trust works well by taking advantage of the tax break called annual gift tax exclusion. You need to send your beneficiary's notice of what you have done to qualify for this gift tax. You can apply your annual insurance premium toward this gift tax. In a 1968 court battle, Dr. Clifford Crummey challenged the IRS and won the right to apply his insurance premium toward the gift tax inclusion.

If you own a regular life insurance policy when you die, the insurance proceeds are subject to taxes. For example, Joe Smith, a widower, has an estate worth $3 million. The estimated taxes on his estate are $675,000. He takes out a $1 million policy to pay the taxes, which he owns. When he dies, the policy is subject to taxes of 45 to 47 percent, or $470,000 of the policy pays estate tax. He could avoid this by not owning a policy when he dies. If someone else owns it, then it is not taxable. The primary benefit of this policy is that taxes are saved.

The trustee can purchase a life insurance contract on your life with funds that you provide. If you transfer an existing policy and die three years after transfer, it will be included in your estate. Sometimes, conditions are imposed when you transfer a policy. A taxpayer can give $11,000 to another person as a tax-free gift. This can buy plenty of life insurance.

The trustee will pay the annual life insurance premium. The trustee must notify their beneficiaries in writing that a gift has been made in their name. Your beneficiaries will have the option of withdrawing funds in an average of 30 days. Written notification of your gift to beneficiaries is the so-called Crummey letter. An annual Crummey letter is an essential element of the Irrevocable Life Insurance Trust.

Charitable Remainder Trust (CRT)

Charities serve two purposes — they help disadvantaged people, and they help the wealthy reduce their tax bills. In 1969, the U.S. Congress created a bill to help charities increase revenues for their causes. The trust allows taxpayers to reduce estate taxes, eliminate capital gains, claim an income tax deduction, and benefit nonprofit organizations. This trust is called a Charitable Remainder Trust.

These trusts are irrevocable and provide for two sets of beneficiaries. The first set is the income beneficiaries, which can be you and your spouse if you are married. The income beneficiaries receive a set percentage of income for life from the trust. The second set of beneficiaries is the charities or nonprofit organizations you name. They receive the principal of the trust after the beneficiaries pass away. Even though this trust is irrevocable, you can change the charitable beneficiaries at any time. In certain cases, you can serve as trustee and retain control of all assets inside the trust.

Due to the fact that the assets are for a charity, you do not pay any capital gains tax on this trust. These taxes can range from 10 to 20 percent on the assets growth. These are ideal for stocks or property with a low-cost basis but high-appreciated value. It allows you to sell your assets without the tax, which passes at full value to trust and family members. The amount of income depends on the percentage of payout you choose and the amount in income the assets generate. The IRS states that the CRT must distribute approximately five percent of market value of assets to be a valid account.

Many people use this trust to help with retirement planning. By setting one up in peak earning years, you can contribute in a variety of ways like zero coupon bonds, non-dividend paying growth stocks, or variable annuities. By letting it grow and not using money, you can have income when you retire. There is no limit on how much you can contribute. It is considered outside your estate by the IRS, and because of this, you can save 48 cents on every dollar. Because these accounts benefit a charity, they qualify you for an income tax deduction. Average deductions range from 20 to 50 percent against your gross income.

Trusts vs. outright gifts

Trusts protect your assets from your creditors and children while you are alive. An outright gift is open season for anyone to try to get a piece of the action. With a trust, you can serve as trustee with your family named as successors. Then you can control and invest assets as you see fit. Once you give it away, you lose control, and the person who has it may spend it all that same day. Trust assets will not count against you should you need to apply to Medicaid. The state cannot go after your trust assets after you die to try to recover the money paid for your medical treatment.

A trust protects assets from claims should your children get divorced. A gift is often spent or is out of your control once it is given. It saves income tax for your children and permits income to be distributed to you for life. It permits backdoor distribution to members of your family should that ever be a necessity. A trust does not increase the Medicaid look-back period as an outright gift does. Previously, gifts were better than trusts, but now the law proves the opposite.

The drawback is that trusts cost money to prepare, as they can set you back $1,000 to $2,500 in preparation fees. It takes time to understand exactly how they work. You will have to open a separate account for the trust. You will need a federal ID number for the trust, and a separate income tax must be filed each year.

Your trustee

If you leave money in a trust, your trustee is responsible for distributing and dealing with the details of the trust to your beneficiaries. They may need to collect estate taxes, invest money, pay bills, file accounting, and pay beneficiaries. Choose a person who can deal with your beneficiaries easily, and a bank or trust company should be appointed as a backup. It is hard to decide whether to use a professional or family member.

There are pros and cons of appointing a family member. It can be good if the person has time and wants to do the job. They may not mind family conflicts and want to see the trust work effectively. The drawback is that your family member may lack the expertise to do the job. Trustees can be long-term, but relatives, banks or trust companies are frequently not. Family members can fight, making it hard to carry out terms of trust for the trustee.

Choosing an institutional trustee has pros and cons as well. You can expect to pay for these services, and it can be costly for a small trust. Banks are impersonal and may not take an individual interest in your trust or how it does. So you may want to talk to other members involved in the trust to see what they think.

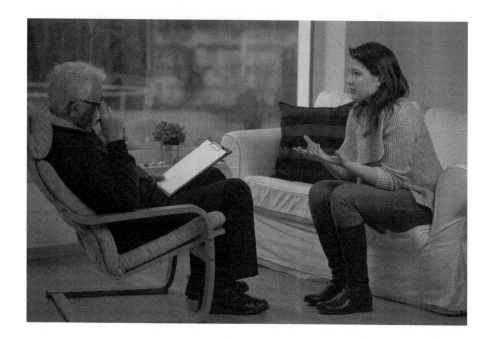

CDs

A CD is short for Certificate of Deposit. This investment is a savings certificate issued by a bank in the form of a promissory note with a fixed maturity date. The maturity date is the date upon which the principal amount of the note is repaid to the investor. The note also contains a fixed interest rate, which means that interest rates on the borrowed amount cannot be raised. Much like an equity-indexed annuity, a CD restricts access to the funds for a certain period of time; in this case, until the maturity date of the investment, which is typically between one month and five years after the initial investment. Likewise, early withdrawal from a CD carries a penalty, usually equal to an established amount of interest. The two types of CDs available are:

- Small CDs

- Large CDs

Small CDs are notes totaling less than $10,000 and carry minimum investment requirements. Large CDs can total as high as $250,000, but no larger because of the cap limit required by the Federal Deposit Insurance Corporation (FDIC), which insures it. CDs can be useful to individuals trying to lower their assets, because it forfeits liquidity for a higher return at some future date. Long term CDs yield higher interest rates compared to shorter term CDs, so if you decide to use CDs, it depends on what you are looking to do with your assets and your money. The main drawback to a longer maturity term is that interest rates may increase while your money is not accessible, which means you will not be able to transfer your funds into another CD with a higher yield. To combat this, investors recommend CD laddering. In other words, instead of buying one large CD, buy a number of smaller CDs that mature at different dates. That way, you have access to cash at frequent intervals, and you have the flexibility to decide when and where to invest if you find a CD with a better interest rate. A classic CD ladder would look something like this:

- $2,000 in a 12-month CD

- $2,000 in a 24-month CD

- $2,000 in a 36-month CD

- $2,000 in a 48-month CD

- $2,000 in a 60-month CD

In this scenario, you would have interest earned at the end of a 12-month period, which you could reinvest while CDs in the 24, 36, 48, and 60-month period mature with greater yields. Twelve months after that, you have yields from the 24-month CD, which you can reinvest into a CD with a higher interest rate. CD laddering creates an ongoing cycle that allows you access to your money and provides the flexibility to reinvest in better deals, which essentially circumvents the limitations highlighted by the CD with longer maturity dates.

Guaranteed Bonds

A guaranteed bond is a type of debt instrument that can be bought and sold between two partners that guarantees principal payment by a third party if the issuer defaults on the payment. Most guaranteed bonds are backed by:

- A local authority

- A bond insurer

- A private group entity

- A government authority

Bonds are issued by these groups when they need immediate capital. You are essentially lending these groups money, and in return, they periodically pay you interest along with the interest at a maturity date. Unlike some annuities or CDs, bonds carry an inherent default risk in its maturity date, which means that you may never receive the principal back and lose the periodic interest payments. However, the third party guarantee offsets this risk and the guarantee means that most of these bonds yield lower interest rates than non-guaranteed bonds. In order to obtain a third party willing to back the guarantee should the issuer default on payment, the bond issuer has to purchase bond insurance. However, doing so enhances their bottom line because it increases their credit rating to AAA, the highest rating on the performance scale. The credit rating itself becomes the insurance because the rating protects the portfolio if the bond issuer goes into default.

The bond market is the largest securities market in the world and provides investors with limitless investment options. The bond issuer offers an annual interest rate known as a coupon, and a time frame that it will promise to repay the principal amount that you loaned to it. The interest rate is usually determined by the current interest rate environment, which allows the coupon to stay competitive with comparable bonds. The length of the maturity date may also determine the amount of risk involved in the sale. As in other asset protection tools, the shorter the maturity date, the lower the risk. Issuers understand the increased risk in a maturity date with a longer term, and will therefore offer higher interest rates to attract buyers willing to dabble in high risk and high reward.

Any bond you buy will be bought in the secondary market where its price and yield determine its value. If interest rates rise, you receive more yields from interest. If interest rates fall, so do your yields. Long-term bonds can be extremely valuable, because older bonds that were sold during higher interest rates can be sold at premium on the secondary market because their coupons are higher.

The key to buying bonds is knowing how much the bond's price will change when interest rates change. This is measured by something called duration — the weighted average of the total number of coupon payments over a period of years. Duration is what investors use to calculate risk and compare bonds with different maturity dates. If you are looking into asset protection, investors commonly purchase bonds as a measure of diversification with other assets. Bonds are also attractive as a means of preserving capital and receiving interest at a set rate that is often higher than short-term savings rates.

FROM THE EXPERT: *Michael Guerrero*

There are a lot of different asset protection strategies. I work with about 50-60 cases per year. I can say, without a doubt, each one has been unique. While there's a set of strategies you can use, there's never a one-size-fits-all approach. It's understanding the situation and adapting to it using what you know about each state, their personal situation, their goals. the realm of possibilities are using spousal protections, using trusts, annuities, and caregiver agreements as ways to protect and/or ensure eligibility sooner.

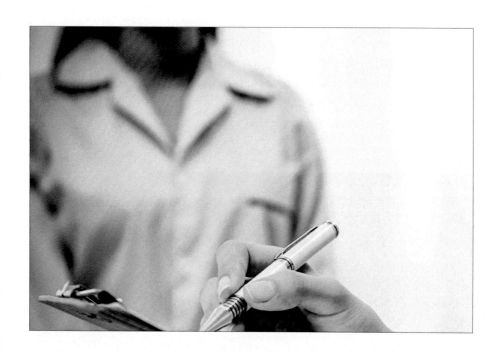

Chapter 5

Asset Protection Strategies — Wills, Deeds, & Your Home

Often, it is not enough to have a will to protect your assets from Medicaid. Now you need more. There are different types of wills that can be prepared by an attorney. A will is a legal document that tells how a person's property should be handled when they die. A will should be written to express the wishes of the person requesting it. Married couples can prepare wills that address inheritance tax protection and the issue of long-term healthcare. By making arrangements, you can insure your spouse will have quality arrangements and medical care.

A well spouse can take action and make sure that if something happened to them, all assets can pass into a Special Need Trust for the ill spouse. All assets will be protected; then the person can apply for Medicaid. A holographic will is one written without witnesses, but few states recognize these wills as legal. Oral wills are also recognized in few states and only in compelling situations like impending death. A self-proving will is one that has been witnessed and signed. It has all formalities required by state law. It can have an attached affidavit signed by a notary public.

A formal will is used in probate. It is put in writing signed by the person making the will and another witness.

Wills

A will should state that you are of sound mind when you sign it. The names, birth dates, and locations of all children, relatives and friends in the will should be stated clearly. You should talk with a lawyer about whether to name stepchildren or illegitimate children in the will. This would be to avoid claims that might come up if you leave them out after your die or even before this.

Appointment of a guardian for any children or stepchildren should be addressed. Consult your lawyer to discuss whether you should have a separate lawyer for your finances. A detailed list of who will inherit specific items of property is often included. Some states have separate lists kept with the will so it can be updated periodically.

The division of property should be fair. Sometimes making provisions through a testamentary trust for minors and those that waste money is a good idea. When heirs have the same name, they must be clearly identified with numbers to tell the difference between them.

Do not put your organ donor wishes in your will or funeral arrangements; most wills are read after the funeral. Only describe the assets you wish to leave to your heirs, but not all of them. It is advisable to try to avoid inflexible instructions like selling all assets; leave that to your executor and heirs. Finally, avoid ambiguous wording as much as possible.

Burial instructions are often included in a will. It is a good idea to have them written up in a separate statement that can be accessed. You may want to have a copy of burial instructions in a separate place.

The will should be kept in a safe place like a safe-deposit box in your home or at the bank. If you keep it in a box, you will have to arrange for an executor to have access to box after your death. Some states put a freeze on the box when you die.

Oral will

Oral wills are spoken to a witness instead of being written down. It is often used by someone who feels there is not enough time to draft and write a document. Frequently, armed service members in active combat make an oral will; fellow soldiers serve as witnesses for the will. This is one type of oral will that most probate courts will recognize. This type of will is not normally recommended due to the possibility of fraud and misinterpretation.

Deathbed will

A deathbed will is often drafted when someone faces death. They are often hard to prove legal and most often challenged by family members. The person can be of sound mind when facing death. They are supposed to be witnessed by two or more people.

Holographic will

Holographic wills are informal and handwritten. Not all states will recognize this sort of will. They must be signed by the person making the will and another witness. They are frequently used when something unexpected or tragic happens. A probate court often finds them invalid.

Self-probating will

Self-probating wills are considered timesavers. When the will is created, a witness signs a statement that the person creating the will was of sound mind. These documents are important because without them, the witness would have to testify in probate court. These wills are created with an attorney and are the least likely to be challenged in court.

Living will

A living will is a written oral statement of medical care about what you specifically do and do not not want when you become unable to take care of yourself and make decisions. It is called a living will, because it takes effect while you are still living. A healthcare provider or good attorney can help you prepare this document. It will help you control what you want to happen when you are ill and cannot speak for yourself. This may never happen, but it is good to be prepared.

Do not confuse this with a *living trust*, which is used to hold and distribute a person's assets. A living trust is used to avoid probate, and it varies from state to state, so you may want to have a lawyer prepare yours. Many lawyers who practice estate planning provide living will and healthcare power of attorney preparation in one complete package.

You may want to talk with your doctor about the type of medical treatments you would refuse if you were in a coma or vegetative state. He or she can answer any questions you may have about these medical procedures.

Living wills by and large describe life-prolonging treatments that you and the doctor do not want to use. This is in the event you suffer a terminal illness or are in a vegetative state. It only becomes effective when you no longer are able to speak for yourself. In many cases, your doctor and another medical person would have to certify the living will in order for you to use it.

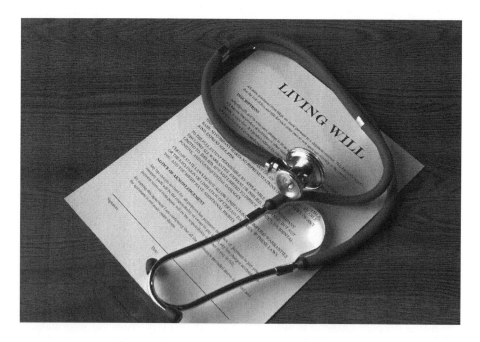

Be sure to talk with your doctor and the person you put in charge of your living will. Keep it in a place where you know it is safe but accessible for others in the event that they need a copy.

Because it is a complex document requiring someone who understands the law, draft a living will with a lawyer specializing in elder law. Your signature and a few witnesses are normally a standard requirement for a living will. In some states, your signature must be notarized to make the will legal. Some states do not allow you to use your doctor or relatives as witnesses. Once the will is completed, give a copy to your doctor, family members, a member of your religious community, the hospital you use, and the nursing home (if you live at one).

Here is an example of a situation that requires a living will:

> Bob was 65 when he had a fatal heart attack at home. He was rushed to the hospital and hooked up to a machine. He was in a vegetative state but was kept alive by these machines. His wife, Mary, wanted him disconnected. However, his parents wanted him to stay on life support, because they believed he would eventually get better. He never made out a will, so no decision could be made for him by any family member. He was unable to make any decisions, which left everyone in a procedural limbo. Needless to say, the cost of his care escalated, and the debate over whether or not to keep him alive caused family members unnecessary stress. If he had a living will made, this would have helped the situation.

If you were in a nursing home permanently and suffered from a stroke after the age of 65, a living will would give someone you trust the power to do what you want with your healthcare. You might be sent to the hospital and then hooked up to a life support machine even if they could not save you. If you have no living will, the system can drain your finances and control your fate. A living will is a good idea for anyone concerned about the big picture with healthcare. It gives someone you trust the power to make decisions for you when you no longer can.

A Health Care Surrogate Designation

A Health Care Surrogate Designation, similar to a living will, is a document naming another person as your representative to make medical decisions for you if you are unable to make them for yourself. This can include instructions about any treatment you do not want.

The designated surrogate can be any competent adult that can make healthcare decisions for you during a time of incapacity; they should consult with your healthcare providers. They only make decisions for the person who made the living will. The decisions are based on what the person directed them to do or would have made themselves if they could. You can designate an alternative surrogate if the first or original person is unable or unwilling to assume the responsibility. A copy must be provided to the healthcare surrogate, and unless a termination date is given, this will remain in effect until the person with the living will revokes it.

The living will and healthcare surrogate can be revoked at any time using a signed and dated letter from the maker. It is important to tell your physician that the living will and surrogate have been revoked. For instance, you can direct the person to donate your organs after death or not to allow you to be kept alive by life support if you are technically dead.

An *anatomical donation* is allowing death donations of all or part of your body. This can be organs and tissue donated to persons in need or to a healthcare facility for training purposes. Organ donors can donate through driver's license renewal or state ID application, or you can put it in a living will.

When planning or making advanced directives, you should ask surrogates if they agree to be responsible for your health decisions, and give them a copy after they sign the legal documents. They should know where the documents are located should they need them. You also can use an attorney to do this.

Set up a file for advanced directives and paperwork. Some people keep them in a bank safety-deposit box. You can keep a card or note in your purse or wallet with information on the safety-deposit box.

Deeds

Survivorship deed

A survivorship deed is used when husband and wife purchase property together. It can be used in other situations. This deed can allow owners to avoid probate upon one person's death, but when the second dies, the property will be subject to probate. It is not suggested as a deed to be used between parents and children unless a lawyer is consulted first. If you want to divide the property equally among several people, this is the wrong deed to use. It can be used if a relative wants to name another co-owner of a home or property. If you have a deed made up long before you apply for Medicaid, the deed should not affect your eligibility. If you have a deed made up before you apply to avoid having your home or land factored in, that may count against you.

Joint owners with rights of survivorship

The most common method of avoiding probate and passing on property after your death is joint ownership with rights of survivorship. There are two common forms of joint ownership. One is called tenancy by the entirety. If husband and wife own the property, then neither can dispose of nor sell the property without the other's. When one spouse dies, the entire property passes to the other spouse. Creditors who have a judgment against one spouse cannot collect a judgment by seizing property.

The other is a form of joint ownership, allowing for survivorship rights between or among two or more people. It is not necessarily husband and wife. The result is the last surviving joint owner receives the full ownership. The difference is that any of the parties can give away their share by selling or giving away their interests. Common forms of property this relates to are autos, bank accounts and real estate.

An advantage of this is that property passes to the surviving co-owners automatically. Often, only a death certificate is needed to deal with the property. Joint bank accounts offer a married couple convenience and flexibility clause. Funds are immediately available if one spouse dies or is incapacitated. These arrangements are suitable to married couples, especially if someone wants to remain living in the house.

One of the disadvantages of joint ownership is loss of control over property. Another is a problem with getting rid of the property or obtaining loans. Serious legal problems and an increase in the cost of probate can occur. Costly and cumbersome conservatorship proceedings and disagreements between owners that may cost in terms of time and money are also negatives of this ownership.

Joint tenancy is a way to own property together. Each state has their own rules by incorporating the following guidelines:

- Both parties must receive ownership rights at the same time.

- A unity of title means both persons are on the same deed or document as owners.

- Both tenants must own equal shares of the property and both tenants have rights to occupy, enjoy and use the property.

Lady Bird Deed or Enhanced Life Estate Deeds

Most families own property they want to give or pass on to family members. One way is to add their names to the deed on your house and land. This method can be full of problems and red tape.

Another way is to make a Lady Bird Deed, which is also known as the Transfer on Death Deed. It works when the owners or grantors deed the property to the children. They reserve a life estate for themselves with the option to sell the property at any time if needed. The deed means the grantors still own the property. The grantor can sell the property at any time. If the grantor never sells the property, it goes to the grantees.

The Lady Bird deed has many virtues. It bypasses probate for real property. It does not result in capital gain and is valued on what it is worth on the day of the last grantor's death, which is called stepped-up value.

It does not open up the property to creditors because grantees do not have much interest until the grantor has passed away and only if they never sold the home. It allows them to sell the property at any time if needed for medical purposes.

The deed is named after Lady Bird Johnson, the First Lady, who inherited property from her husband from one of these deeds. It is not used that much because trusts are more expensive then wills and more complicated to set up. This deed avoids a costly probate process. The states of California, Texas, Ohio, Florida, and many others now use this deed.

Sometimes, a Quit Claim Deed is made to make it easier for the family. The problem with this is the owner would not be able to mortgage or sell the property without the consent of the beneficiaries. It is often used to avoid probate.

The deed is also called an Enhanced Life Estate Deed, a mechanism to bypass the probate process. The husband and wife retain the right to live on the property for life. They control what happens to the property so at any time, they can sell or revoke the deed. Individuals or couples who want to simplify the transfer of their property upon death while retaining full control of it while alive can use it. Medicaid eligibility will not be affected, as long as the intent to return to the home is demonstrated.

This deed is good for a woman who wants to pass on the property to her children without probate but remain in control of her estate.

Do not put your children's names as joint tenants with rights of survivorship. If you do this, the property may not be protected from creditors, so in effect, you can lose your lifetime protection. You might be disqualified from Medicaid should you have to go to a nursing home. You may have to pay a heavy gift tax and you may not be able to sell your home if you choose to. A person can sell or change the deed without notifying her beneficiaries.

Beneficiary deeds

A beneficiary deed will disqualify a person who needs long-term care from receiving Medicaid benefits. When it comes to real estate, this deed does not allow the person to name a beneficiary in most states. Transferring property requires a probate hearing along with the expense.

Transferring real estate at death is easier now in Colorado; it is called the beneficiary deed. It is made by the property owner and recorded in real estate records. The deed can be revoked at any time before the death of the owner.

There are many issues to consider before making such a simple deed. Any-one who thinks they will apply for Medicaid should not make this type of deed. It will disqualify the person from Medicaid as long as the deed is in effect. If a parent leaves the property to three children and one dies, then the two left will inherit the property. It does not sever joint tenancy. It cannot be used to avoid the debts of the deceased.

It is cheaper than a living trust, and has no gift tax liability. It can be changed at any time or revoked. Since it is not transferred until death of the last owner, the value of the property remains in the estate of the deceased for estate tax purposes. When there are several beneficiaries, they will own undivided interest in the property. It can make the property hard to manage or control.

Other deeds

Joint tenancy with rights of survivorship is a document or deed where two people own half of the property equally. When one dies, the other acquires the right to the property completely; it is by right of survivorship. To establish ownership, the other party or survivor must get a certificate of death that is transferred out of probate, which makes it easy and profitable. The survivor is not required to record the deed, so it gives some privacy against those who might object to the transfer. When one tenant or owner dies, creditors lose their rights against the property. It is an irrevocable deed and is taxable as a gift when it is executed.

An enhanced life estate deed is another name for a ladybird or joint tenancy deed. The owners retain the right to mortgage, sell, give a gift, or cancel the remaining interest at any time. Couples who want to attain full control over their property should use this type of deed.

It is a mistake to add children as survivors. If you deed property to children and retain life estate, your home may not be protected from creditors and you may not qualify for Medicaid should you go into a nursing home. Your heir may have to pay a hefty gift tax on the property or assets. You may not be able to use your home to pay for the medical care you need.

The state of Massachusetts has a deed called a declaration of estate of homestead. It is filed with the Registry of Deeds in the county where your home or property is located and can protect property up to $500,000 of the value of a primary residence per family. A sole person commonly files this deed, and if family members own the house with you, they have homestead protection. It protects your home against attachment of levy or sale to satisfy debts. The property or home of persons 65 or older is protected, and couples filing jointly will be protected despite marital status. A letter certified by licensed physicians or the Social Security administration must be included when you register for declaration of estate of homestead. Only one spouse or person in the home under age 62 can file for this deed.

Liens imposed by the state for Medicaid are exempt from homestead protection. The state will not file a suit especially if the spouse is alive. If the surviving spouse is also on Medicaid, the state will file a claim for reimbursement for the entire amount of Medicaid benefits paid. The rules are complicated, so it is good to get legal advice.

Estate recovery trends in individual states

States have different policies on estate recovery, and some are more aggressive in seeking money from estates. Michigan tends to ignore estate-recovery programs, much to the anger of taxpayers. The Deficit Reduction Act of 2005 enforces penalties on individuals who purposefully hide assets with the intention of qualifying for Medicaid.

In Pennsylvania, "estate" refers to all property and all probate estate property; this means all real estate and personal property of the deceased person. Life insurance is subject to claim and also deposit and patient-care accounts.

Since Georgia instituted an estate-recovery program on May 1, 2006, more than 100 patients have returned home or left the nursing homes they were in because of fear of losing their homes. Others have dropped Medicaid coverage or home-care services. Massachusetts has instituted a more aggressive program with liens against homes to claim an estate when a Medicaid recipient passes away.

Georgia and Michigan were the last two states to adopt estate recovery plans. Of course, this practice is causing heated debate, because the state claims assets from estates of Medicaid applicants. Many live in nursing homes and then pass away while owing Medicaid money. Many states have been slow to adopt the rules, because it forces them to collect money from families that have used up money on long-term care. Some people feel this plan turns Medicaid into a predatory loan for those over 55.

States with limited budgets seek to recover some of the money lost on the Medicaid program. The goal of Medicaid estate recovery is not to bankrupt people but to receive some money back.

Utah recovers money from the estate of Medicaid recipients providing there is no child blind, disabled, or under the age of 21. Recovery takes place only after the death of the Medicaid recipient and the surviving spouse. The maximum amount of recovery is the amount paid for medical expenses for a recipient age 56 and older. Your home is exempt for Medicaid eligibility but not from estate recovery.

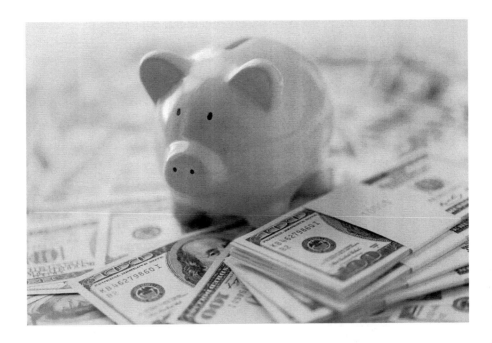

Utah proceeds with estate recovery by having the Office of Recovery Services contact the heirs after the death of the Medicaid recipient. The organization may record a lien against real property of a deceased recipient to obtain estate recovery. They may file a claim with the court for the amount of medical assistance provided.

Florida estate recovery will not file a claim when there is a surviving spouse, the recipient is under the age of 55, or a minor or disabled child lives in the estate. The state only claims the amount paid on behalf of the Medicaid recipient for services rendered.

Florida law requires any representative of an estate to notify all creditors. Medicaid is a creditor of an individual receiving benefits from the Medicaid program. State agencies such as the Vital Statistics and Social Security offices often share information about deaths of Medicaid recipients with state agencies. This is the way the states know to file a claim on a Medicaid applicant's estate.

In Indiana, when a Medicaid recipient dies or has an estate, they will file a claim against the estate to be reimbursed for services paid on behalf of that person when they are aged 65 or older. This includes services to those under 55 if made after October 1, 1993. Claims include all services provided to Medicaid recipients.

All assets are subject to estate recovery. Many assets not counted for Medicaid eligibility may be counted in estate recovery. Assets not subject to recovery are life insurance or annuities. The first $125,000 of jointly held property with right of survivorship in Indiana is not subject to estate recovery. Real estate used for the support of a surviving spouse is excluded. Personal effects, keepsakes, and ornaments of the deceased are often excluded as well.

In 2007, the U.S. Court of Appeals was asked to approve a request by the state of West Virginia—an exemption that would allow homeowners to retain $50,000 of their home against Medicaid claims to recover the cost of nursing home care. Federal Medicaid officials denied that request, resulting in many West Virginians refusing to apply for Medicaid.

In Pennsylvania, Medicaid applicants are often told about the estate recovery program by caseworkers during the application process. Only medical assistance received after the age of 55 and for specific types of services are subject to estate recovery. The state seeks reimbursement for nursing facility, home and community, hospital, and prescription drug services.

New York requires recovery from the estate of Medicaid recipients who are 55 or older. It can recover from the estate of the spouse, except if the spouse is still living in the house or has a disabled child under 21 living in house.

Oregon has tough new Medicaid estate recovery policies for long-term care. The new rules can collect money from your estate after you die for Medicaid costs for long-term care in a nursing home or for home services. A nursing home spouse used to be able to transfer the house to the well spouse to shield the assets from Medicaid use. Now, if someone transfers the house in the five-year look-back period, the house would become a countable asset. It will be hard for people to protect their homes from estate recovery if they need Medicaid in the future.

What to Do With Your Home

Your home is one of your biggest assets in Medicaid because it is excluded while you are living there, but can become the subject of collections when the Medicaid recipient dies. There are different tactics available to make sure your home is not taken by the state when someone in the family is either on Medicaid or will be applying for it.

If you are permanently in a nursing home and no relative lives in your home, you must make an effort to sell the home by listing your property with a realtor or selling it privately.

Transfer your home with a special power of appointment. Here, you transfer the ownership of your house to someone else while reserving your right to redirect the house to a different person at a later time. You could exercise this power during your lifetime (by a deed) or at your death (by a will), subject to certain limitations. With this tool, the state would be unable to go after the house either during your lifetime or after your death, though you would lose the legal right to live in the house.

Keep it, sell it, or transfer to kids?

People over 65 ask this major question when thinking about a nursing home or passing on real estate and money to family members. Determinations should be made about the home. Have a registered real estate agent appraise the home for value to give you an idea of what it is worth.

Keeping the house has its benefits in that you will have a place to live and not have to acclimate to an unfamiliar place. Although there is some inheritance tax, more often than not it is much less than income tax owed.

The drawbacks include an inheritance tax of the property upon death of the owner. If the owner becomes ill, there will be no lien and the state does not require it to be sold. Yet, upon death of the person, the state can claim the estate for the amount used for Medicaid. They cannot collect if another person owns the estate.

If you sell your home, federal income tax allows $250,000 exclusion of the gain on the sale of principal residence. It allows $500,000 for a married couple. The proceeds can be given to the intended heir without the payment of a federal gift tax. If the donor of this money applies for medical assistance, the applications must report any gifts and amount given within the five years preceding the application.

This can be a serious problem because Medicaid applicant will have no money unless the transfer took place more than five years prior to the eligibility. The older person has to live somewhere and may need to use proceeds to rent accommodations.

When you transfer the deed to your kids, they become liable for maintenance, taxes, and insurance. There will be no inheritance tax on the property for one year.

The gift or transfer will result in a five-year period of Medicaid ineligibility. Giving the house away and reserving the right to live there will result in an inheritance tax on the full value of the house on the date of death. Another problem with transferring the deed is that if the person dies, or is involved in divorce, creditors can claim the property.

Joint ownership

Joint ownership refers to two parties owning property together. Property may apply to a residence or business. If one owner dies, they do not have to go to probate. This often applies to real estate owned by a married couple, like a home. A parent can jointly own a home with a child.

If the parent has only one child's name on the deed for joint ownership but wants to divide the property among other children, this presents a problem. If the parent dies, the child whose name is on the joint ownership does not have to carry out the parent's wishes. He or she will be the sole owner of the property.

A remarriage can result in your children being disinherited under a joint ownership. Children's creditors may try to collect on their share of the property. Your property could end up with someone else owning it rather than your intentions. A co-owner could transfer you shares to someone else without your knowledge or approval. If anyone is in a high-risk profession, the house is subject to the risk of that profession. The gift tax and estate costs could be extremely high. It is awfully hard to remove a co-owner's name from a deed without their approval.

Joint property allows the surviving spouse to do whatever they want with the previously jointly-owned property during their lifetime and ultimately leave it to anyone they wish at death, regardless of your desires. This can be an issue in second and third marriages.

You can transfer the house and property to your kids, but this is a disqualifying factor when you apply for Medicaid. You will have to take the cost of your home and property and divide it by the cost of a nursing home per month in your state. This will give you the amount of time you may be disqualified from Medicaid. When you deed the house to someone, you no longer own it; you lose control over what happens to it. Your kids can kick you out, make you move, or even sell it if they choose.

Add children's names to the deed

Adding your son or daughter's name to your deed means they own half of your home, and own it outright upon your death. It frees property from getting tied up in probate court.

Though unless you are wealthy or use it early, it will not save you much in estate taxes. Since they own part of the home, creditors can come after it as an asset. Once the name is on the deed, you have to have the agreement of the child to get the name off the deed. A minor child on the deed needs someone appointed by the court to represent them before you can do anything with the home. Minors cannot transfer or refinance property. You will have to pay for legal fees to get representation for your child. In short, do not add minor children on the deed of your home.

To get an adult or minor child's name off the deed, you can file a quick claim deed that states say they have no interest in this house. You may run into a problem if the child wants money from the ownership of this property. What if your child runs into drug problems or tax trouble? You may have to sell your home to settle the debt for them; which is one of the drawbacks of this type of ownership.

Transfer to a sibling

The transfer of a home to a sibling of a Medicaid applicant will not incur a penalty if the brother or sister was living in the house at least one year prior to the date the applicant was admitted to a nursing home. Another factor to remember is that the sibling has an equity interest in the house. This means that some percentage of the home was gifted to them. This can be as small an amount as 2 percent.

A transfer of a home to the child of the Medicaid applicant who is under age 21, blind, or disabled will not cause any penalties to the applicant. If you can prove you made the transfer of a home for reasons other than qualifying for Medicaid, and the transfer falls into the five-year look-back period, it may be excused. You must present to the state clear and objective evidence that the house was transferred to the applicant for reasons other than qualifying for Medicaid.

Life estate

A life estate is a form of interest in a piece of property that allows the person with it to retain a full interest in the property until their death, but gives legal title to another person. You can purchase life estate in your child's home if you move in, for instance.

If your parent moves into your home, this can be another way to protect your parent's assets. Parents sell their home and move into your home. The child will sign a deed transferring a percent of their home equal to the amount of the parent's estate, and the parent transfers cash to the child in the amount equal to the value of that interest. They must live in the house at least one year after the deed is signed. Otherwise, the purchase of interest is called a gift to the child and Medicaid can count it.

Jane and Ted purchased a home for $700,000. Ted's mother, Mary, has declining health and needs assistance during the day. Mary sells her home and moves in with Jane and Ted, writing them a check in exchange for a life estate. If after one year she has to be moved to a nursing home, interest in her house will not be counted since it is considered an interest in a personal residence, and such an interest is almost always excluded as an asset.

Transfer to children while keeping life estate

You can transfer your house to one or more children in the house but retain your life estate. This is the right to possess the property during your lifetime. When you die, the title passes automatically to the child or children to whom you deeded the interest in the house.

You have the right to live in the house during your lifetime. After death, the estate is subject to taxes and the children who own the home will receive a stepped-up tax basis. If you are on Medicaid, the state may be able to force a sale of the property collecting the value of the life estate. After you die, it goes to your children without going to probate court.

You can give your children 1 percent interest and own the home together as joint tenants with the right to survivorship. It may not hurt if you apply for Medicaid because a transfer of 1 percent is not much of a gift and would be not be taxed much on penalty. If you decide to use joint tenants, consult an experienced lawyer that really knows the Medicaid laws.

Purchase a joint interest in a child's home

Sometimes parents will purchase a joint interest in their child's house. They must reside in the home at least one year before moving into a nursing home to have this valid and not counted as a gift transaction. The longer the parent resides in the home after purchasing a joint interest, the better it looks to Medicaid when someone has to apply for benefits.

It can reduce the estate tax liability and removes valuable assets from your estate, thus further lowering your estate tax liability. Parents who purchase a home jointly with a child share the home's value. An alternative is a joint purchase, but not a typical joint ownership. One party purchases the life interest and the other purchases the remainder. There is no gift tax as long as the property is valued and each party paid his or her appropriate share.

Life interest is just that, interest for life. Interest terminates at the person's death, as there is nothing to transfer and thus nothing is subject to estate taxes. Whoever owns the remainder of the interest is now the owner of the property.

In cases of joint purchase, nothing is transferred at death. Commonly, when family members are parents to a split interest transaction, the remainder interest is valued at zero. The purchase is deemed a gift from the life tenant to the remainder interest holder.

Child moves into your home

If it so happens your child moves into your home to provide round-the-clock care, Medicaid will allow the applicant the right to transfer the homestead to the caregiver. The rules require that the caregiver live in the homestead for at least two years prior to the applicant's admission to a long-term care facility. A physician's statement must document that the care would have otherwise required long-term care. The two-year period must be made immediately before the nursing home entry. A stay in an assisted living center would break the continuous period.

There are caregiver agreements covered by Medicaid for the elderly who do not want to move out but need care at home. There is often a relative willing to move in to care for them. Caregiver agreements are written contracts in which a relative agrees to care for someone for an agreed amount. Often, the home and person will be investigated; a criminal background check may result.

Living with a parent can cause changes in the family roles. You will find it stressful and there will be differences in sleeping, eating, and social patterns that may be difficult to adjust to. You should talk about the move before you do it and be honest to look at the pros and cons. Do you want to devote the time needed to help your family member, or would you resent it?

A program in Massachusetts allows family members to stay at home and be paid to care for vulnerable elderly relatives who might otherwise have to go to a nursing home. Caregivers receive up to $18,000 per year for home-based care. The savings are excellent compared to the cost of semi-private nursing home. They are supported by a team of professionals through regular home visits and telephone contact.

With help from a lawyer, Jane recently signed a contract to help an elderly aunt. She will be responsible for taking her to doctor appointments, cleaning her apartment, authorizing payment of her bills, and helping with laundry; she is paid for her services. This service can reduce the size of an estate and eventually help the relative qualify for Medicaid assistance. It can reward the child who does spend most of the time caregiving, while other siblings may not have time or the inclination towards this duty.

Working out the terms of the contract can make the process less painful, as no one feels they are being taken advantage of. The contract spells out a specific course of action, and the caregiver is compensated financially. There is an uptick in this service.

Medicaid most likely will not disqualify you for having these contracts with your family. Contracts that pass the Medicaid guidelines have to follow some rules. These rules are: you cannot pay the caregiver an inflated price just to spend down assets, they can make the current market rate for those services by contacting agencies that provide these services and getting estimates, services can vary from meal preparation, laundry, cleaning to providing transportation, caregivers have to pay taxes on services and only work a few hours per week, and some states have to offer caregiver training and education.

Parent moves in to the home

The financial burden or taking care of an elderly parent in your home is time consuming and stressful. The pros and cons should be weighed seriously before making a commitment to caring for anyone in their home or yours. There are many factors to consider in this decision.

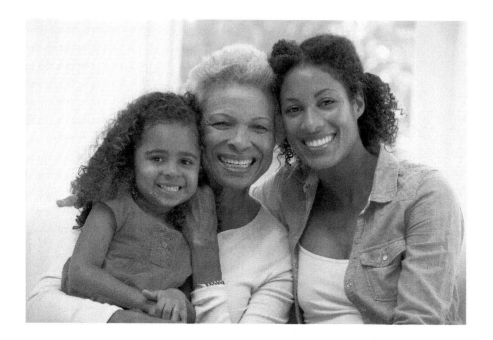

Emotional issues are one area to consider:

- Do you and your parents have a good relationship and get along? If you never did, then living with them will not work for anyone.

- How do your parents get along with your children and partner?

- Can you emotionally deal with becoming your parent's parent?

- Do your children respect the elderly person and enjoy their company?

- Can you include them in your social activities and other routines without too much stress?

- Does everyone in your family want the elderly person to move in?

- Most elderly relatives need care when they move in. Can you provide them with that care or find someone else to help you?

- Does your job allow you time off to take them to doctor appointments?

- Do you have time to take them to visit friends or the senior center where they can socialize with other people?

Living arrangements are exceedingly important as well:

- Do you have the space needed to accommodate your parents?

- Do you have an extra room or addition that will give them some privacy?

- Is it possible you will need some special equipment like wheelchairs, walkers, or grab bars in the bathroom?

- How safe is your home for the elderly?

- Do you have any loose steps or areas that need railing or ramps?

- Do you live in a steep hilly area where getting in and out of the house is difficult?

- Do you have an area of the house where you can go for some privacy?

- Do you have the money to accomplish any renovations needed?

If you live in a small house with three children, it will get more crowded and congested. A larger home works better for having your elderly parents move in with you. It is important to have the space for them so they feel welcome and have some privacy. You need to set some rules so your parent or relative respects the other members of your household. If you truly resent having to live with your elderly parents, then it is better not to. However, you should still find another alternative.

Financial considerations are another area to contemplate:

- Does the elderly person get some assistance so they can contribute financially to your household and their own needs?

- How much will you have to pay out of your own pocket to help them live there?

- Will your brothers and sisters or relatives help with the financial end?

- Can you discuss money with your parent so they know what is expected of them?

Some universal rules for living with an elderly parent that apply to all families:

- Establish house rules for everyone to follow. This will help with meals, privacy, and other important issues. Set limits on both the elderly person and the children so they can get along with each other. They need to respect each other's privacy and schedules.

- Make sure everyone has some privacy. If this means adding another bathroom or having a schedule worked out, do it. If you have to rearrange the décor or buy a divider for a few rooms, do so.

- Work out a budget that includes letting the elderly person contribute to household expenses. Never assume; discuss finances before the person moves in so hidden expenses do not surprise you.

- Let the elderly person help around the house and be as independent as possible. This is good for their self-esteem. Encourage them to have their own interests and hobbies.

- If the person has health problems, keep the doctor and emergency numbers handy so that most family members know where to find them. Discuss this with your family so that when an emergency arises they will know where to look and what to do.

- Safety is important for everyone. Make sure your parent does not leave medications around if you have younger children. Toys lying around can be hazardous for anyone with walking difficulties.

Taxes on the home

Your home should be included in your taxable estate. For anyone applying for Medicaid, owing estate taxes is not a real problem. Your estate must be over $2 million and anyone with that much money does not need Medicaid.

There is a tax rule that says if you retain the right to live in your house for the rest of your life, it will be included in your taxable estate. This causes the house to get a new income tax value equal to the date of death value of the property. This eliminates any capital gains if and when they sell the house immediately upon your death. The right to live in the house does not have to be in writing; it can be an agreement.

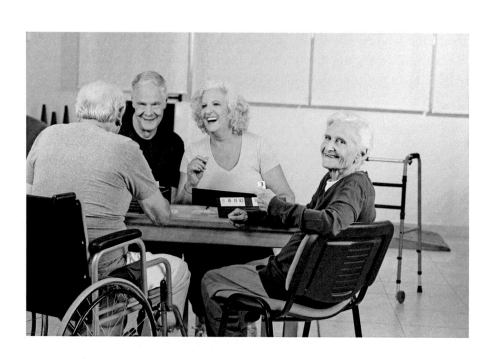

Chapter 6

Long-Term Care Options

Home Care Programs

Many states are adopting home care programs in an effort to cut Medicaid spending. It is a new trend, and many of the programs are slow to get started. Depending on what state you live in, there are different types of home-based Medicaid programs. Other government programs that do not come under Medicaid fund some state programs. We will discuss some of the new programs offered in several different states.

The Adult Family Care program in New Hampshire was designed to move about 500 seniors from nursing homes back into the community. The seniors will live with their families or others paid to participate in the program. This program was designed to cut Medicaid spending by paying individuals to take seniors into their homes and provide non-medical and personal care. There are two programs located in Manchester and Nashua. The providers for this program are relatives, friends, or strangers who are approved by the state to participate in the program.

The program began slowly because it takes time to approve licenses and do background checks on individuals who want to participate as caregivers in the program. The program is designed for seniors healthy enough to live with someone in the community. They do not need long-term nursing home care due to severe or chronic medical problems. The elderly participants have a registered nurse evaluate whether they can be moved into the community to live. The nursing home costs about $140 per patient, per day. This program pays $60 per day for food, rent, transportation, and the caregiver's time. Not many caregivers are participating in this program so far, but it is a start.

It is important to have residential alternatives for the elderly in their remaining years. For some elderly persons, a nursing home alternative is a good choice.

The Alabama Choices Program began in 2007. It was a program that gave seniors a monthly allowance for determining what services they need to live independently. The seniors use the money to hire someone to help with household tasks or use the money for medical equipment or supplies. Financial counselors are available to help participants understand and manage the money for this program. Alabama is one of the first states to add this program. It gives seniors control over the home services they use.

Colorado provides some home care services under the HCBS-EBD Home Community Based Services and Elderly, Blind and Disabled programs. The services provided under this program are homemaker services, non-medical transportation, personal care, respite care, electronic monitoring, and home modifications. This program is paid under the Medicaid program.

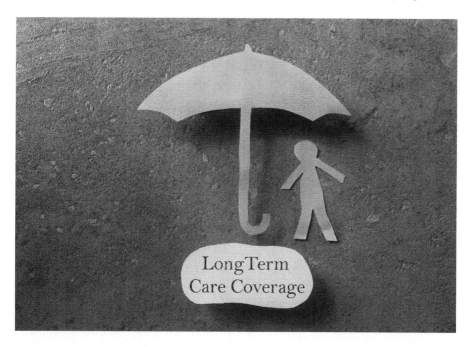

Connecticut has a program called the Connecticut Home Care Program for Elders. It is for elderly persons at risk of going into a nursing home. To qualify, you must be aged 65 years or older and meet the financial qualifications of the program. To apply, you must call and request the home care application form from the Connecticut Department of Social Services. If you are in the hospital or a nursing home, the staff can give the forms there. The form will give you the details and asset guidelines to help you decide if you qualify for the program. You will have to have a health screening and have your eligibility determined by the department clinical staff.

If you qualify for the program, a case manager will determine what services you need to help you live independently. These services can be:

- Homemaker services

- Visiting nurse services

- Home health aide

- Delivered meals

- Someone to help with chores

- Emergency response system

- Medical services

Minnesota has two different programs under the home and community based waiver program for the elderly. One is called the Alternative Care program. It is a program for persons 65 years or older who need assistance but not long-term medical care. It pays for trained caregivers, home delivered meals, and household chores. The program prevents or delays an elderly person's admission into a nursing home. This program covers a variety of services for the elderly at home. The second is called the Elderly Waiver program for those over 65 who need to be in a nursing home but prefer to remain living at home. These clients need medical assistance to live comfortably at home. The program covers visits by a skilled nurse, home health aides, companions, personal assistants, and also home delivered meals, and equipment modifications.

New Mexico has a new program called Money Follows the Person. This program enables the money to follow the elderly person from the nursing home back into the community. They must be evaluated to determine if they are able to make the transition. It is a new program that has had a slow start. The program gives the elderly person a choice of living in a nursing home, in the community with their family, or at a foster home.

In Ohio, many elderly patients prefer to live independently in their own home and near relatives and friends. Many entered nursing homes but the Passport Medicaid Waiver Program has helped some elderly patients stay at home. The benefit of the program was it gave them a choice. Applicants are screened and then provided with the different long-term care options available in their community.

The second part is simple; once the elderly person is found eligible, a worker will put together a package of homecare services that suits the person's needs. The person must be 60 years or older to participate. They must be fragile enough to require nursing home care and able to stay safely at home with the permission of their physician. Some of the services provided are meals, food, transportation, and housekeeping.

More than 27 states received Money Follows the Person grants. This new program allows the states to transfer nursing home residents back into the community. Connecticut has received $24.2 million to create a system to move nursing home residents back into the community. The program also uses Medicaid dollars for more flexibility, giving seniors more choices for living arrangements. Even 24- hour homecare may be an option for some under this program. This program's funding covers assisted living centers, the family home, or an apartment.

Florida's Cash and Carry Program allows clients to hire their own help and use the funds to buy equipment or supplies. Grace, an 82-year-old woman living alone, has many health problems and was never was satisfied with the help she received. Through the Cash and Carry Program, she chooses the homecare service that will help her and uses the remainder of the money to buy things she needs for herself. She is more satisfied with this program than any of the other Medicaid programs she has used before.

Assisted Living Centers

Many seniors and elderly persons live in assisted living centers. More than one million elderly persons who have mild memory disorders and chronic medical conditions that do not require constant medical care live in these centers. Assisted living centers offer seniors a place to live independently, yet provide services like meals, housekeeping, transportation, social activities, emergency call systems, personal laundry services, and 24-hour on-site staff. Some centers are covered by Medicaid, but many are not. Some assisted living centers offer limited medical assistance with medication supervision and other simple medical services.

Assisted living centers are called continuing care retirement communities, personal care homes, and retirement home for adults. Some of these communities have libraries, theatres, game rooms, laundry services, gardens, and transportation for shopping. Many centers covered by Medicaid have terminated their contracts, making residents move to another facility after living there for several years. Many assisted living centers prefer private pay clients as opposed to Medicaid clients.

Assisted living centers are a good alternative for those that need assistance but not 24-hour nursing home care. Families can live nearby and check or visit with the elderly person at many assisted living centers. Many families often live within 15 to 20 miles of the assisted living center. The cost ranges from $1,500 to $5,000 per month. Some expenses are covered by long-term health insurance policies and Medicaid. Many assisted living center do not use either.

Here are some guidelines to follow when checking out an assisted living center for a family member or friend. Ask some of the following questions:

- What is the building and surrounding area like?

- What type of meals do they serve the clients?

- Do the meals meet healthy dietary restrictions?

- How large is the facility and does your relative prefer small or larger settings?

- What are the visiting hours?

- Is the site odor-free and clean in terms of appearance?

- Are pets allowed to live with residents?

- What is the cost of the center, and do they have any financial assistance for residents?

Look carefully at the services and activities of the assisted living center before committing a family member, and ask the following questions:

- Do they encourage socialization and have facilities for this?

- Do the units have phones and refrigerators?

- Is it near a shopping center and other entertainment?

- Do they have religious services or a library?

- Does the kitchen have a refrigerator, stove and dishwashing unit in it?

- Do they have adequate space to store the person's belongings?

What are the financial considerations you must consider? Ask the following questions:

- What is the cost and is a deposit required?

- What services are included in the cost and what has to be paid for separately?

- Is the facility connected with a nursing home?

- Are utilities included in the cost of the monthly fee?

- What types of housing are available?

- Does the price of the assisted living center go up regularly?

Safety is another important issue for seniors. Check some of the following aspects when you visit the center.

- Does each room have an intercom?

- Are there proper safety devices such as lighting, exits for fires, or fire extinguishers?

- Are there handrails, door alarms, and emergency buttons or cords for seniors?

- Are there readable signs on entrances and exits?

- Does it have air conditioning and heating?

- Is it a safe location with doors that are easy to lock?

- Is the facility in a good location?

- Is it near a hospital, stores, a post office, and pharmacy?

Many assisted living centers accept patients who are too ill to truly live there. Before you decide on an assisted living center, make sure your parent or relative does not need long-term nursing care. One assisted living facility accepted an elderly man with dementia. One night the patient climbed out the window when the temperature dropped to 26 or below. He was found dead from exposure the following day. He was not supervised properly at this assisted living center.

Another patient with Alzheimer's disease was accepted into an assisted living center; he developed bedsores and signs of malnutrition after entering the facility for just a short period. These centers are not always equipped to take care of elderly patients with serious physical or mental illnesses. Be sure they have a proper medical staff before enrolling anyone in an assisted living facility.

There was another case where a man raped an elderly woman with Alzheimer's disease in an assisted living center. When you learn the facts about the patients, you will find the man was a mentally ill patient with a criminal past who lived in the assisted living center. Both patients should not have been in the assisted living center because it was not set up to care for either of them properly. They both should have been supervised constantly and extremely carefully. The facility was investigated and found to be negligent to residents in many areas.

It was found that in this facility, patients were often locked in their rooms. Residents were not fed properly and complained of not having enough food. It was found that personal care supplies often ran out and staff used paper towels sometimes instead of toilet paper. They advertised social activities that never took place. The state investigated the facility and found 63 violations, which tells you this assisted living center was not regularly inspected. Cases like this have been found in Florida, California, Virginia, Ohio, Texas, and other states. That is why it is important to learn as much as you can about a facility before you commit anyone you know to stay there. There are many satisfactory assisted living centers, but some are not.

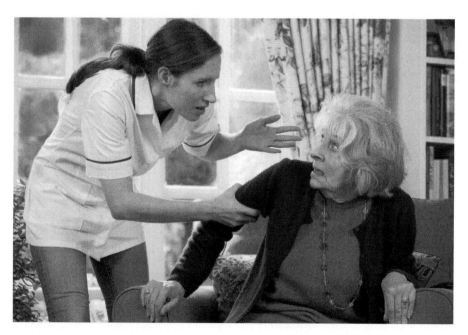

Seniors who need 24-hour long-term medical care should not be enrolled in an assisted living center. Anyone with dementia or Alzheimer's disease who needs constant supervision because of memory problems is not a good candidate for the assisted living centers. Serious medical conditions like chronic heart disease, kidney problems, and diabetes, where seniors need medical and diet supervision, may not be safe in assisted living centers. It is important to know the medical staff is on-hand to treat these diseases.

Most assisted living centers must meet certain federal and state guidelines. When you check into one for a family member or friend, find out if they are certified by the state. They should offer your client privacy, autonomy, and choices. There are a variety of laws that pertain to assisted living centers about services delivery and discrimination. The building must meet certain safety requirements, zoning laws, and landlord-tenant requirements to be in business.

The Informed Choice Legislation was passed in Oklahoma in June 2007. It states that residents can remain at an assisted living center as long as a physician says it meets the criteria of care the patient needs. It also states that family and the patient must all agree that the needs can be met through the assisted living center and the community. This gives the elderly person a choice where to live and does not force them too early into a nursing home.

The state of Tennessee allows Medicaid assistance for its assisted living centers. This will give many elderly a choice of where to live. More than 40 states have adopted the waiver program that allows some seniors to use Medicaid dollars for assisted living centers. The cost of an assisted living center is about half of that of a nursing home. Many state and federal officials view it as a more appropriate setting for the elderly.

In 2006, California decided to test assisted living centers as an alternative to nursing homes with residents who did not need strict medical long-term supervision. It allowed Med-Cal, which is Medicaid to cover the costs of some residents in California assisted living centers. This would save the state money in Medicaid spending. Arkansas, one of the poorest and most rural states in the U.S., provides financial aid for assisted living using Medicaid dollars for poor, elderly clients that qualify. It has a large population of persons over 65. This state lured assisted living developers using tax credits, streamlined regulations, and flexible Medicaid reimbursement rates. This has lowered Medicaid spending by about 10 percent in this state.

Last July, Ohio enacted a Medicaid assisted living program. It was expanded later to include those seniors already residing in assisted living centers. The proposal was passed because nursing home operators now often operate assisted living centers. Medicaid covers about 240 of the 33,000 assisted living centers, so this percentage is low. Only 58 of the 280 eligible facilities accept Medicaid residents. The rates are not what they should be, therefore fewer facilities want to participate in the Medicaid program.

Adult Day Care

If you are a caregiver or have an elderly relative or friend who lives alone, adult day care might benefit both of you. It is a planned program of social and health-related services offered during the day for seniors. The program provides meals and snacks as part of the program. Seniors who do not need 24-hour care are often good candidates for adult day care centers. They must be mobile but can use walkers, canes and wheelchairs. They must not be incontinent. Some adult day care centers take patients in the early stages of Alzheimer's disease. Many programs do not provide the necessary medical assistance, so this should be considered before signing someone up for the program.

Some of the activities provided in the adult day care centers are arts and crafts activities, musical entertainment, sing-alongs, birthday and holiday celebrations, book discussion groups, movies, and theatre productions. Some provide transportation to the center, blood pressure, and eye screening. This type of adult day care has limited medical assistance and supervision for patients. The average age is 72 years and older, and about two-thirds of the program participants are women. Also, one-quarter live alone, and three-quarters live with a spouse or other family members and friends.

Family, clients, and charitable donations pay for the programs at these centers.

Follow these tips when deciding on whether an adult day care center is right for your family member. Find out how many years the business has been in operation and if they are licensed and certified by the state. This is important because then they will be checked regularly for code violations. What are the hours, and do they provide transportations services? Evaluate their menu to make sure they offer healthy food choices and not just snack foods.

Visit the adult day care center and check to see how clean it is:

- Does it smell?

- Is the staff friendly, and how do the other clients seem?

- What is the cost, and what is expected of you if you are the caregiver?

- Do they have any volunteers that assist the staff?

- Are the furniture and facility safe for the elderly?

- Do they have grab bars and handicapped access for those less mobile?

- Are you able to use wheelchairs easily in the facility?

- Is it roomy or cramped and overcrowded?

- What are the credentials of the staff?

The advantages of an adult day care center include that it gives adult, working children a structured place to leave their elderly relative or friend. It helps ease the guilt of putting an elderly person in a nursing home unnecessarily. It gives the caregiver a break from a 24-hours-a-day job that often has no relief. Many programs do not provide family members assistance with medications, physical therapy, or occupational therapy.

Sherrie's 96-year-old mother fell and had to have hip replacement surgery. She had to move in with Sherrie and her husband, Wayne. The constant care of her mother caused Sherrie fatigue and depression. Her mother agreed to try an adult day care center near their home. She enjoyed the social activities and the yoga exercise program. It relieved Sherrie four days a week so she could work, clean the house, and be with her family and friends. The program gave her mother a life of her own. That can be the advantage of an adult day care program.

The purpose of an adult day care program is that it provides a structure for elderly patients. Even if they can handle living alone, it is healthy to spend time with other people in a structured environment. Even low-income elderly clients deserve to be able to have access to this type of program.

The Daily Living Center, an adult day center in Tennessee for low-income seniors, was afraid they might have to close their doors due to budget cuts. Their clients decided to address the problem by holding a garage sale. It was a place for the elderly clients to have a meal and socialize. The program was spared the budget cuts, but the effort the clients put into saving the center shows how meaningful some of these programs are. It was specifically designed for low-income seniors in Tennessee.

The schedule at the Daily Living Center is as follows: Seniors arrive about 8:30 a.m. for breakfast. When the weather is good, they go for a walk around 9:15 or do an exercise video. They are provided with lunch, play games, and have a rest period. During the day, the seniors are always busy doing activities that are good for them physically and mentally. The program provides the necessary structure for these seniors.

Maryland has an adult day dare program that is funded by Medicaid. Care is provided at medically approved facilities to those who qualify, including some seniors. Under this program, adult day care offers many services including medical assistance. The funding for Medicaid and adult day care centers varies from state to state. The Center For Medicaid and Medicare began a pilot program in 2007 that allows some money to go to adult day care. Under the program, Medicare gets a five percent discount on what they would pay for patients' home health costs.

Tennessee Options For Community Living Programs will pay for adult daycare and also the Medicaid waiver program. The demand for adult day care is increasing by 5 to 15 percent yearly. There are about 400,000 elderly clients served nationwide by this service. Medicaid pays for low-income elderly clients to go to the adult day care program. Many have too high of an income to qualify for this program, however. Many states are passing legislation to get Medicaid-funded day care options for the elderly.

Budget cuts in Medicaid threaten some adult day care programs for the elderly. In California, due to the expense, the governor has proposed a 10 percent rate cut for some programs, including those that treat Alzheimer's patients. He also wanted to delay Medicaid checks to some adult daycare providers. Cuts in this program will have devastating effects to the community members it serves.

There are different types of adult daycare centers. Some just provide elderly clients with a place to go with structured activities and are licensed by the state to operate. Others provide medical services needed for those with chronic long-term illnesses.

Adult Day Healthcare Options

Adult day care health centers are for elderly people who need a place to go and get treatment for chronic illnesses. They provide medical supervision in an adult day care setting. They provide a program that keeps an elderly person from going into a nursing home. These centers frequently have several medical professionals on staff to oversee the care of clients that attend the facility. They often have a doctor, registered nurse, social worker, occupational therapist, and physical therapist. The medical components require that the facility have qualified medical personnel on staff, which is the difference between an adult day care provider and adult day healthcare provider.

Adult healthcare centers must offer rehabilitation services with adequate room for physical and speech therapy. They must have adequate room for equipment with written treatment plans and assessment. They should have nursing services for monitoring medications and know how to use restraints properly. Nutrition services must meet health and sanitation regulations of the state. These centers must provide psychiatric or psychological services with plans for care. Recreational and social activities must be designed for individual participants. Transportation to and from the centers is often provided. There are some centers that provide special care for patients with Alzheimer's disease.

Alzheimer's adult health day care centers should provide exercise and social activities for patients. There should be a registered nurse to supervise health and medications. There should be assistance with personal care. The facility should work with the family, physician and staff to coordinate treatment. There should be transportation and good nutritional meals planned. In some states, Medicaid often pays for qualified elderly patients to attend these centers. These centers should be licensed by the state you live in. Most often, if they are funded by any state or federal program, then they are licensed to provide services.

When Helen, an 81-year-old woman with Alzheimer's disease living alone, realized she could no longer cope due to confusion and memory loss, she turned to her healthy elderly family friends for help. Mike and Loretta, a married couple, let her move in with them. They could not stay at home with her all the time, as they had other family and job responsibilities. A local day healthcare center provided Helen with the structure and care she needed during the day so she could live with her friends without being a burden. She spends the day doing simple exercises, participating in social activities and eating nutritional meals. Mike and Loretta are free to work and spend time helping in the community.

These centers play a big role in relieving family members of the stress of taking care of someone with Alzheimer's disease. It also delays the process of having to put the person in a nursing home by giving the patient a place to go to get medical and social treatment. The patients are getting therapeutic and social care and giving the caregivers needed respite.

It is shown in a study by the state of California that many elderly patients with chronic illnesses use adult daycare health services. This includes the fragile elderly who suffered from strokes and falls. Elderly patients who have arthritis, heart disease, Down syndrome, and brain injuries, often use adult day health centers. Some communities will develop a particular day care health center to help a specific medical population.

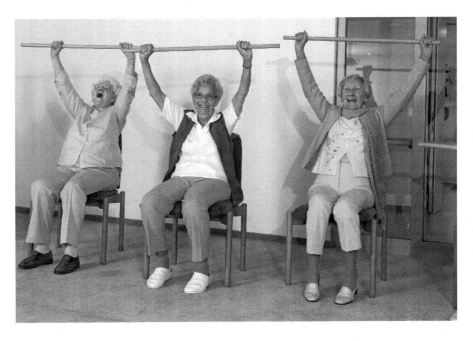

Here are some questions to ask when looking for a quality day healthcare center for an elderly family member or friend:

- Is the center licensed?

- Do they have a qualified medical staff?

- What are the hours of the program for the clients?

- Does the program accept clients with dementia, Alzheimer's disease, limited mobility, or incontinence?

- Do they have special services and medical staff for these medical problems?

- What is the cost of the program per day or week?

- Are there any discounts for lower income clients and does Medicaid, Medicare or private insurance cover the cost of the program?

- What services are part of the program?

Check on the kinds of activities the center offers for clients:

- Are there arts and crafts programs? What about exercise programs?

- Do they provide assistance with bathing and going to the bathroom?

- Do they have dietary services and regular meals?

- Do they perform medical assessments, medications management, and adequate medical treatment?

- Do they have physical or occupational therapy?

- Are activities varied and geared to the client's interest?

- Do residents have input and help plan activities?

You should also ask questions about the staff and how they handle daily operations:

- What are the qualifications of staff members?

- Can caregivers or family members stay at the center with the client during the day?

- Is there a section for sick or ill clients to sleep or sit?

- How do they handle medical emergencies?

- How does staff handle difficult behavior?

Always check the physical environment of a facility. The physical environment should be clean and free of odor. Ask yourself the following questions:

- What is the temperature in the rooms?

- Is it well-lit and quiet with room to move around?

- Do noise levels stay moderate?

- Is smoking allowed?

- Does it have comfortable furniture with tables and chairs to sit in?

- Overall, is the building and grounds well cared for?

- What is the staff like?

- How do they interact with other people?

- Does the food look and smell good, and do they have a varied menu?

- Does the center meet state and federal fire codes?

- Are there emergency exits, fire extinguishers, and built in sprinkler systems for fires?

- Is the center wheel chair accessible with ramps?

- How do they handle patients wandering off?

- Does the center offer transportation for appointments?

- Is there an extra cost for transportation available for non-medical appointments?

- Is transportation wheelchair accessible?

Adult day care in the United States serves approximately 400,000 elderly persons. The average daily cost is about $61 per day. It is about half the cost of daily nursing home care. It will become a viable alternative to nursing homes as the years go on—that's why you need to ask any many questions as possible.

Taking Care of Your Parents or Elderly Relative

Recent changes in Medicaid make it harder to qualify by giving away money or assets to your child. Under the new rules, if you have a legal contract to help your parents out as a caregiver, this will not be counted as a gift. Many elder lawyers now draft caregiving contracts between children and the parents. Some are between other family members or friends.

The caregiving contract should specify the chores the elderly person wants you to perform. One woman set up a contract with her elderly aunt with the help of a lawyer. The contract specified that she would help with transportation and other household chores. All contracts should specify hours and how many times a month or week the service will be provided. Fees paid should be competitive with other homecare services. It helps with estate problems down the road to have a legal contract. The contract has to follow strict guidelines to pass Medicaid authorities. Consult an elder care attorney to draw up a caregiving contract for you.

In 2006, a program called Caregiver Homes in Massachusetts provided up to $18,000 per year for caregivers to help elderly relatives live at home. It was covered under the Medicaid Enhanced Foster Care Program. It allowed family members and friends to give full-time caregiving to fragile elderly relatives or friends. It gave the elderly patients and their families an alternative to nursing homes care. Participants must be members of Mass-Health, also known as Medicaid, and need assistance with at least three daily living activities. Caregivers are supported by a team of professionals led by a registered nurse who is the case manager. They are given specialized training through the program and connections to other social service programs. Each caregiver is carefully screened and receives payment for their services to the family member.

There are many family members who live with an elderly relative and take care of them. Many are not paid, but may be qualified for this program and not realize it. For those who want to take care of their parents, this is a good option.

Susanne takes care of her elderly 88-year-old father at his home. Her mother died about a year ago from heart disease. Through this innovative program located in Massachusetts, she helps him bathe, dress, and take medications. The program pays the individual caretaker or provides the participant with foster care. Individuals willing to take someone into their home to live must pass strict state requirements. The program targets low-income seniors in an effort to give them the option of living at home. There are similar programs in the state of Minnesota.

Caregiving can be frustrating and lonely, but for some, it is incredibly rewarding. Sometimes, it is a way to repay a parent or relative who helped you become the person you are today. Sometimes, it is a deep commitment to family that makes one take on the challenge. Elder care inspires some people to create or lobby for changes in the laws. They never would have done this before, however caring for a loved one inspired them to seek change for that person. Even if you cannot handle the caretaking because it is too physically or mentally draining, you can seek help. Never feel you have to do everything alone. You can find many wonderful programs and services through a little research.

If you are contributing financial support to your elderly parent, you may be able to get a tax break. First, if you are supporting your elderly parent to get a tax break, you will have to put them on your income as a dependent. To get this tax break, they will have to meet the following conditions listed below.

- The person's 2007 income must be less than $3,400. Income from Social Security or disability does not count against the total.

- Any money from other sources of income such as pension benefits, interest and dividends from investments, or withdrawals from retirement savings plans cannot be claimed.

- You must provide more than half of your parent's cost of living expenses including housing, food, medical care, transportation and other necessities.

- Your parent does not have to live with you. IRS publication 501 has a worksheet for you on this topic. Pick it up and talk with your accountant or financial expert today. Please check with your accountant regarding these conditions.

There are different types of caregivers. An informal caregiver is commonly a spouse, child or friend of the person. The person does not normally receive payment for services such as shopping, transportation and cleaning. Below are some tips on finding caregiving services for your elderly relative or friend.

Nonprofit organizations and churches often run soup kitchens and food pantries. They collect canned and dry food items so people can go to the soup kitchen to get food. Home-delivered meals and group meal sites are available to seniors 60 years or older. This is through a federally-funded nutrition program. There is no fee for these programs, but donations are accepted.

The group meals sites, sometimes called congregate sites, are located throughout the community. They offer opportunities to meet new friends and interact with others. The centers sometimes offer nutritional screening and diet counseling. Home-delivered meals, known as Meals on Wheels, are available to the elderly who cannot make it to the meal site. Volunteers deliver a well-balanced lunch each weekday.

There are many small businesses that provide caregiving services to the elderly. They employ people part-time to help seniors with meal preparation, house cleaning and other chores. This offers people viable part-time employment and also provides a needed service. Over the next decade, the needs of the elderly will provide careers in nursing, social work, computers. Those working with the elderly often find it a rewarding job.

If you decide to have your mother or father or relative live with you, it is not easy. Caregiving regularly falls to women but more men are now involved in the process. The caregiver's well-being can only be maintained by finding a balance between that role and other areas of your life; it is important to have time away from that role. Learn to pick and choose what you do and do not do. If your parents need transportation, perhaps you can find some alternative methods of transportation like buses for seniors or hiring someone to drive them. Their health insurance or Medicaid may cover it.

There are many organizations now for caregivers that support the person caring for elderly parents, relatives or friends. They provide articles, a listing of services that can help, or respite care for the caregiver, which gives them up to date information. Some nonprofit organizations even offer volunteers who help the elderly living at home alone. If you plan to be a caregiver, your local agency on aging may offer workshops and support for this role. Some even provide caregiving training workshops.

Local Agencies on Aging in New York offer caregiving workshops. They offer caregivers a chance to meet others in similar situations. One of the workshops offered is Men Making Meals, a cooking class for male caregivers where they learn to prepare simple nutritious meals. Other seminars are How to Balance a Checkbook and What's Under the Hood, a basic car maintenance course. So if you are taking on the caregiving role, your local office of the Agency on Aging can be a good source of information and support.

When your parent becomes ill and unable to take care of themselves, the first instinct is to have them move in with you. This is understandable, but not always the best move for your parents or yourself. Consider some of these factors before you take the plunge.

Do you and your parents get along well enough to be together full time? Is your home properly equipped or is it small and cramped? Do you have the financial ability to help them out, or are you struggling yourself to make ends meet? What does your parent want? Often, they do not want to live with a child because of lifestyle differences they are undoubtedly aware of.

Try the arrangement out on a trial basis for a limited amount of time such as one month. Be clear that this is a trial basis arrangement. You can even try the arrangement out for a week. Weigh the following considerations if you decide this is the right path for you.

Relationships are an important part of how families function. How will your siblings and relatives feel about you taking your mother or father into your home? Can you all sit down and discuss the subject rationally? Does he or she have friends that will visit him or her or are you their only social contact? What are the limits of care that you can provide before you need outside help?

How will you adapt your home to your elderly parents? Do you have adequate space for them to stay, such as an extra room or addition? Do you have the assistive devices they may need like grab bars, raised toilet seats, and ramps? If not, can you afford to add them to your home? Does your mother have a pet, and do you have room and the environment to take it on?

Financial considerations must be thought through. Stress over money can make caregiving more taxing.

What will be the financial arrangement? Will I expect rent from my parent or relative? How will my siblings feel and will they contribute to the parent's living expenses? Do I have resources to meet the bill with another person living in my home? Am I comfortable helping my parents bathe or changing an adult diaper? Is there respite help available for me if I need it?

There are caregiver groups that meet to discuss the problems and joys of caregiving. These groups can be of help if you choose to be a caregiver. It is healthy to talk with other people who share similar problems. Often, you can share information and solutions to your difficulties. You will find that caregivers come from all walks of life and have a common bond helping out a family member. Members can share positive methods of coping with a difficult situation.

If you are considering groups, look at some of the following factors to decide if you want to join the caregiving group. Do you want a formal group that gives training seminars or a more informal group that meets to talk about issues? It is best to pick a group that meets your needs.

A group that has been in existence for a few years or even more is a good idea. A group that continues to look for new members is a positive sign that they are active and a good resource for caregivers. Who does the group focus on, the elderly or a group with a specific disease or age range? It is important to find a group that deals with issues that are relevant to your situation.

Finally, look for a group leader who has caregiving experience, so you will learn something new. If there are no groups where you live, do you have time to consider organizing one yourself? Some groups offer training in developing support groups so you can learn from experienced people.

The advantage of a support group is that it is a place to share feeling and experiences. You realize you are not alone and isolated, and others share your experience. You can often get assistance and help, as others know something you may not. Some nonprofit organizations that help the elderly have support groups for caregivers.

Those caring for someone with dementia and Alzheimer's disease will find many support groups that address the issues. It is vital to find a group that respects your choice and offers help with doing the job you want. It is important to find a group that offers options for those facing caring for a family member. A group that knows about respite care and services for these patients is helpful.

Sometimes, the support group is the only support you will get for caregiving. Your family might not be supportive for reasons ranging from not having enough time to personal problems that interfere. Sharing and caring with the group can become your lifeline in coping with the courageous choice you made to care for your family member.

Call your local area agency on aging or senior center for referrals. Hospitals and community groups often can assist. Fraternal organizations such as the Elks, Moose or Eagles often offer assistance. If your relative or friend is a long-time member, assistance can include home visits and transportation. They often offer transportation to and from senior centers. Veterans frequently can find a variety of services available through their local Veteran's Administration Hospital.

Alternative Healthcare

Considering other forms of therapy that some doctors recommend is another option. Dr. Andrew Veil and Dr. Dean Ornish advocate natural rather than synthetic medicine. They offer programs regarding low fat diets, vegetarianism, meditation, group support and yoga. Some insurance health plans cover some forms of alternative medicine.

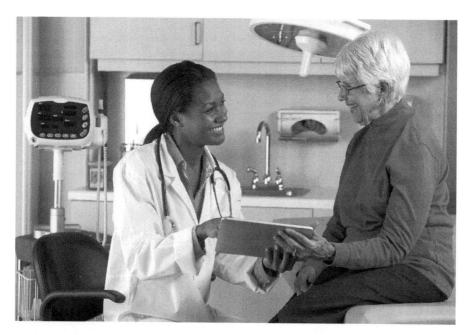

What are some of these alternative healthcare options? Some are massage therapy and deep tissue bodywork, vitamins and herbal supplements, vegetarianism, yoga and meditation. This form of medicine treats the whole person, making lifestyle changes that help with the overall illness.

Alternative medicine should not be used as substitute for regular healthcare. It can be used in addition to treatment to help with diet, attitude, and overall health.

Talk with your doctor before you use an alternative health plan. They often work with those not suffering from long-term chronic illnesses that need traditional treatment. Alternative treatments often can be used in addition to regular treatment for illnesses.

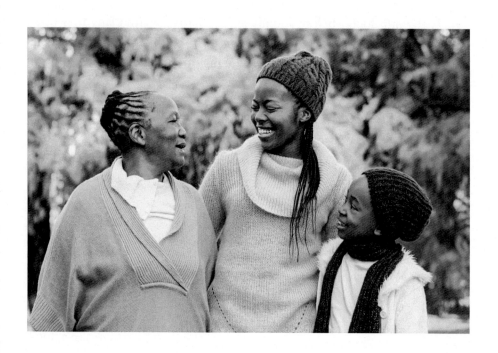

Chapter 7

Single vs. Married — Resources

Determining Value of Assets

The value of an asset is the amount of money you can get for it in the marketplace, minus any debt. A home is a major asset. What you can sell a home for depends on the geographic region and the economy. A home worth $530,000 might sell for $550,000 if the market is right. Some assets are counted when determining Medicaid while others are excluded. Knowing the difference can help you act wisely with your assets.

Any asset that can be changed to cash is frequently considered a countable asset. A checking account, savings account, or having cash in the house in a vault are considered countable assets. Certificates of deposit, stocks, bonds, and mutual funds also are countable assets, as are IRAs and other kinds of retirement accounts, life insurance that can be converted to cash value, annuities, and all autos except the first car. Extra buildings, machinery, and leisure items such as campers, boats, livestock, horses, and tractors may be countable assets.

Countable assets

The general rule of thumb about countable assets is that if you can spend it or convert it to cash, it is considered countable income under Medicaid.

Cash, checking accounts, savings, and certificates of deposit (CD) are countable income. Other investments like stock bonds, IRA, 401(k), and retirement accounts are considered countable income. A life insurance cash value is countable if you can convert it to cash and the value is more than $1,500. If you own more than one car, the second, third, and fourth car are countable. If you own more than one truck, tractor, boat, piece of machinery, or livestock, those assets are also countable. If you have additional land that is not excluded, it is most likely countable.

Bank deposits will regularly include savings, checking, CDs, or other accounts in a financial institution. An IRA is an individual retirement account that you maintain at a bank with special rules that allow you to avoid income tax until retirement. Tax laws impose heavy tax on early withdrawal of IRAs. It is undoubtedly a countable asset.

Securities mean stocks, bonds, mutual funds, promissory notes, and other assets. A security is commonly countable unless it has no market value.

Excluded assets

This may surprise you, but there are many assets that are excluded from Medicaid when determining eligibility. These assets are not countable toward your eligibility or your spouse's eligibility. If you are single or married and are determined eligible for Medicaid, the most basic rule is that you can have $2,000 cash; that is the limit. You have to keep your account below this or you could lose all of your Medicaid benefits.

Your home—if you are single and live in the house—is excluded from Medicaid if the equity is $750,000 or less. There are certain conditions that allow the home to be excluded if you are on Medicaid. One is if you will be in a nursing home for a certain period of time and plan to return. Another is if you have relatives who live in the house with you or own equity in the house—a spouse, dependent child, disabled child, sister or brother, or parents. The equity in the home is what Medicaid looks at. For instance, if you and your husband own a home worth $300,000, then your equity in the house is $150,000.

If you are married and permanently living in a nursing home, your home is excluded if your spouse or other relative lives in the house. If you are in a nursing home and the value of your equity rises above the state limit, you can lose your Medicaid benefits. It is important to keep equity in the house below the limits set by Medicaid. The land the house sits on and other buildings are excluded as long as the equity is below $750,000.

Let's say you live alone in the house and plan to return after your nursing home stay. You have been qualified for Medicaid to pay your nursing home expenses. If you are ill and cannot communicate your interest in returning to your house, a spouse or a dependent relative is allowed to communicate your intent to return to the house to a Medicaid representative or nursing home. If you moved from your home to an assisted-living center or apartment, your home will not be excluded as an asset for Medicaid, because it is not your main residence.

What about selling the house? The house would be excluded as long as money from the sale is used to secure residence in another home no later than three months after the sale. Whatever money remains, barring what is invested into another home, would be counted. If your spouse lived in the house, the spouse could keep the money, as that person would be considered the community spouse.

One auto is excluded, and it can be of any value. If the person owns more than one auto or other vehicles, those vehicles are countable at market value. If you own two cars, a motorcycle, and a truck, the second car, motorcycle, and truck, would be counted as assets.

Regardless of their value, personal property defined as jewelry, furniture, household appliances, and computers are excluded from Medicaid. They are items used on a regular basis, items that have been in the family, or items with sentimental value, such as wedding rings, necklaces, and artwork. Some items can be counted, especially if they are collected for investment purposes, such as jewelry, art, and other collectibles.

Funeral and burial expenses are often excluded, depending on the nature of the account. You can set aside about $1,500 in a bank account or trust for a funeral. This money will be excluded as long as it is below the limit and specified for this purpose. For a married couple, each person can have $1,500 in a bank account for funeral and burial expenses.

Medicaid for Massachusetts' residents is called MassHealth. It combines Medicaid and the Children's Health Insurance Program (CHIP), and members may get doctor visits, prescription drugs, hospital stays and other services at little or no cost. Cemetery plots may be purchased for the nursing home applicant, spouse, and any family members. A burial account may be started to pay for any expenses not covered with up to $1,500 each for husband and wife. You can buy a single premium insurance policy to pay for funeral expenses. Assigning the value of surrender to a funeral home makes the asset or value non-countable. Purchasing a prepaid funeral contract or irrevocable trust designated for funeral and burial expenses are acceptable ways to spend down assets. An irrevocable burial contract is not counted in Massachusetts.

Money people pay for their funeral and burial arrangements is excluded, and there is no limit on the amount. You can spend as much as you want on your burial arrangements, even if you do it long before you become ill. If you make arrangements with a funeral home, the money you put aside must be put in an escrow account or trust. Some states require a contract declaring that any extra funds not used for the funeral arrangements be paid to the nursing home or Medicaid. Even life insurance to be used for funerals or burials is excluded. You can prepay for burial expenses for your spouse and children, parents, and siblings. This includes burial spots, coffins, funeral proceeding, urns, and other traditional items.

If a Medicaid applicant is single, IRAs and other retirement accounts are countable assets. If an applicant is married and the spouse is living at home, these accounts are often not counted. Conversely, some states count the IRAs of both spouses.

Properties or buildings used for self-support by applicants normally are excluded from asset inclusion. If you own and operate a small dairy farm, the farm property—including the land, buildings, and storage areas—is excluded. A small business at home used by you or your spouse may be excluded. Be aware that many states ignore this rule, or use the $6,000 (or 6 percent) rule. This means that if you own property not used in trade or business but make money renting it for use by mobile homes, only $6,000 of the property value can be excluded. This is especially true if you make a 6 percent or greater profit on renting land to mobile home users.

The life insurance policy owned by a Medicaid recipient frequently is excluded. The cash value of a policy smaller than $1,500 is not counted. If you want to keep a policy for burial, you might want to transfer the life insurance policy to a family member and have that person pay the premium if it helps with burial expenses.

Unavailable assets

Some assets are not counted, because they are not legally available to the person who is going on Medicaid. What circumstance determine whether an asset is unavailable? This means a person does not have the legal right to use or dispose of an asset—this can be because of a contract, court order, or law. Assets that cannot be sold are unavailable.

In order for an asset to be considered unavailable, you may have to produce evidence that it is not sellable. This can be done by getting experts in the geographic area with knowledge of assets to state in writing that it is not worth anything. For real estate, an actual sale attempt may have to be made in order to prove it cannot be sold. If no offer is received, then that is proof of it being unavailable.

If an asset is owned by more than one person and cannot be sold without the other person's consent, it is often unavailable. If the second person refuses to sell the asset, then it is considered an unavailable asset.

For example, if you are named an heir in someone's estate when they die, then the asset is not available to you until that person passes away. This asset would be excluded. If you own real estate that cannot be sold due to legal problems or other technical complications, then this property would be excluded. A lawsuit that you filed prior to receiving Medicaid assistance where you were awarded money or which was settled long before you filed for assistance would be excluded.

Community Spouse

Federal law protects spouses of Medicaid applicants through what is called a community spouse resource allowance (CSRA). The community spouse is defined as the spouse of the Medicaid applicant, and under this provision, the community spouse does not have to spend down their assets in order to qualify for Medicaid benefits. This provision also increases the likelihood of the Medicaid applicant's eligibility. The resource allowance comes into play when the spouse has to enter the Medicaid applicant into a nursing home. The CRSA is usually half of the couple's resources, minus the resources that are exempt under Medicaid rules.

Before applying for a CSRA, you need to be sure that you or your spouse meets the definition of a CSRA, otherwise you will not be entitled to the benefits. To do this, you must first figure out which assets are exempt, divide that by two, and compile the figures before the date of your spouse's admission into a nursing facility. As of 2016, the minimum home equity limit is $552,000 and the maximum is $828,000. The community spouse's resources must total at least $23,844 and no more than $119,220. Medicaid allows the community spouse a minimum monthly maintenance needs allowance of $2,002.50 and a maximum of $2,980. A community spouse that does not have at least the minimum income is allowed to receive a supplement from the income of the nursing home spouse to reach the allowance requirement. The Medicaid department will allow the community spouse an increase above the minimum—if there is sufficient resident income—by consideration of whether she needs an "excess shelter allowance."

If most of the couple's income and assets are in the name of the spouse applying for Medicaid, the community spouse is entitled to some or all of the monthly income of the institutionalized spouse, depending on what Medicaid determines to be the minimum income level of the community spouse. The minimum income level is determined by calculations based on housing costs. If you feel you need an increase in your minimum monthly maintenance needs allowance provided by Medicaid, you can file an appeal to the state Medicaid agency or obtain a court order of spousal support.

FROM THE EXPERT: *Michael Guerrero*

In some cases, it's going to be very significant for a spouse to have an income stream that is topped up by their sicker spouse. It might be a younger or healthier wife whose husband has been the primary earner because of a lifetime working. They have retirement, they have higher social security income, and she did not. There's something called the Minimum Monthly Needs Allowance. This is like a guaranteed minimum income for a healthier spouse whose partner needs to be in nursing home care.

50 & 100 Percent States

Some states allow the community spouse or person who is not in a nursing home to keep 50 percent of the couple's joint countable assets. This is especially true of married couples that have one person living in a nursing home due to chronic illness. These are known as the 50 percent states. Some states allow the community spouse to keep 100 percent of the couple's joint countable assets up to a certain dollar and not have to contribute the money to Medicaid. These are known as 100 percent states. Each state has different rules, so check with your state office.

The Snapshot Rule

The snapshot rule refers to the date an account of finances is looked at to see what should be counted or excluded, should an applicant eventually need Medicaid. It is regularly the first day of the month a person enters the nursing home. The community spouse should get a resource assessment from a caseworker when a spouse enters a nursing home. This is not the same as applying for Medicaid, but it will determine the couple's countable income. The sooner you get a resource assessment, the sooner you will know where your assets stand with social services.

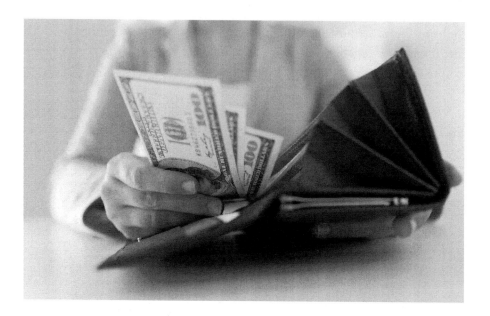

A split transfer offers the Medicaid applicant a method to shorten his or her eligibility period without having to give away all property before a 60-month look-back period. Under the 50/50 split transfer method, the person may give away half the property or assets during the look-back period and retain the other half. The gift is calculated as part of the ineligibility period. The person spends down the retained assets. Often, this cuts the ineligibility period in half. This is a conservative approach to save money on assets. One must plan ahead to do this successfully.

For example, John lives in a state where a nursing home cost $5,000 per month. He has $240,000 in assets. He gives his daughter $120,000 as a gift on June 1, 2006. He applies for Medicaid on May 1, 2010. The gift is within his 60-month look-back period, so he uses $120,000 for his nursing home care for this 12-month or longer ineligibility period.

Purchasing Annuities

Some companies will not issue a policy on someone who is over 85; other companies will go as high as 90. It is important to find out about the company before purchasing any product. Check with the Better Business Bureau, consult a professional, or contact your local chamber of commerce for information. Most often, an annuity can be purchased for a single person in any amount. Another point to remember is that if the policy is based on life expectancy longer than the person purchasing the annuity, then some part of the purchase price will be considered a gift to Medicaid.

It does not pay for a single person to buy an annuity in a state that requires it to be counted or used for Medicaid. Check with your state agency on rules before you purchase any annuity in your state for that particular purpose.

Most annuity contracts do not contain language for or are not written to qualify for Medicaid rules. The monthly payment must be for the life expectancy of the person purchasing the policy. The annuity cannot have any free look-back period in the contract, and the value is agreed to be zero by all parties. The only value is the monthly income it generates. This feature as part of the contract is allowed in 29 states.

Commissions for Medicaid spend down annuities are low, while commissions on standard annuities are frequently higher. They sell you a product, but one that never qualifies for Medicaid. Always work with a reputable qualified elder lawyer and/or senior specialist when you purchase a Medicaid annuity.

Many single elderly persons over 65 are sold annuities that they are told are guaranteed. They often believe they will not have to lose assets to Medicaid. When the elderly person becomes ill and needs to go into the nursing home, they find that the annuity is counted. They often have to sell or surrender the annuity and face heavy costs. They lose their assets, because the annuity never protected their assets. Be careful when you buy a policy; make sure it will help you.

Most payments go to a nursing home or are used for allowable medical expenses. For a Medicaid recipient, an annuity does not benefit the family in most cases.

If your parent is single and owns substantial retirement and savings accounts, it is not to their benefit to buy an annuity. For those who have enough money to pay for their own care, you will get higher quality long-term care than Medicaid would provide. Whatever income they received from an annuity would almost certainly go to Medicaid. So, it may be wise to avoid purchasing an annuity. Remember, if you plan accordingly with the right life insurance policy, you can alleviate the stress involved with paying for long-term care as well as avoid spending down your assets.

Do not forget about the Deficit Reduction Act of 2005 that says if you purchase an annuity to protect your assets from Medicaid, the state must be named one of the beneficiaries for them to not count the annuity. Always consult a good elder lawyer before purchasing an annuity.

A relatively new rule states that any annuity purchased for Medicaid planning must name the state as a beneficiary. The state must be named the beneficiary after the community spouse and a disabled child, especially in cases of Medicaid patients receiving long-term care. The federal law changed the term from annuitant to institutionalized individual. When the community spouse purchases an annuity for a spouse in a nursing home, they must name the state as beneficiary for the remaining payments after the person passes away. The spouse in the nursing home is known as the institutionalized individual.

If there is a surviving spouse or disabled child named as beneficiary of the annuity, the state will have to wait until the death of that person to collect on the debt. If the payments have stopped, then there may be no funds available at the death of the community spouse. It makes sense to purchase the shortest possible term annuity.

If the community spouse enters the nursing home after the nursing home spouse passes away, the state may request to be named beneficiary of the annuity or estate, so it gets the money for reimbursement of the Medicaid funding for the community spouse. The state will only be repaid money for the person who was put into a nursing home at the time the annuity was purchased.

In some states, the payment of the annuity to a community spouse can cause income of the spouse to exceed MMMNA. This will often be used by the nursing home as countable income.

Chapter 8

Elder Lawyers

Elder law is a growing practice and involves much more than just protecting your financial asset. It is a complex area of law that needs experts who understand state and federal regulations that affect the elderly. This applies to Medicaid and other government programs that are designed to help the elderly with long-term care.

It is growing field due to the baby boomers and a large population of elderly born during 1946-1964. This group needs lawyers for themselves and often for their parents. They represent the elderly person in many areas including abuse, neglect, insurance, long-term care, patient's rights, age discrimination, and asset protection.

Elder law deals with the preservation and transfer of assets when a spouse enters a nursing home to help prevent Spousal Impoverishment. They deal with Medicaid, Medicare, Social Security, and disability claims and appeals. Supplemental and long-term health insurance is another important issue elder lawyers face. Disability planning can be another area an elder lawyer can help clients with. Estate planning, long-term care placement, elder abuse and fraud, housing issues, and mental health are all areas that elder lawyers are involved in. Many specialize in certain areas.

FROM THE EXPERT: *Marty Fogarty*

The elder lawyer has to be familiar with everything from "getting my long-term care insurance qualified," "selling my house," and "protecting my assets," to "a regular revocable trust" and "an irrevocable asset protection trust." The elder lawyer has to know more of that. The problem with using a regular estate-planning attorney is that you have fewer variables on the table. If you want to make beautiful music, you can play three notes or 10 notes. 10 notes are going to give you better music because you've got more variables.

When you look for an elder lawyer, look for one who is specialized in the area you are seeking assistance; start with National Elder Law Foundation. It is the only organization certified by American Bar Association (ABA) to certify lawyers in this particular area. Anyone who is certified has gone through the trouble of studying and preparing to specialize in this area, as they have to pass an exam to be certified.

Also, look at the biographical information of the person. Do they have the education and expertise in the area you are seeking? Ask other people if they have heard of the attorney and what they think of them.

FROM THE EXPERT: *Marty Fogarty*

Go to www.eldersmart.net. It's a nonprofit that's going to offer guidance. Don't go to NAELA, which is an organization of elder law attorneys, or to some sort of elder law group, because all it takes to join a NAELA is to pay a couple thousand dollars to an organization. Just because I can pay money and get a sticker on my website doesn't mean I'm any good.

Elder Smart locates services that families need, and it does that in a way that's going to minimize the time that families waste and maximize the kind of "cut to the chase, let's get the plan, let's get this stuff taken care of" effect. If you go to the elder law attorney, and he's a one-trick pony, and all he can say is, "Well, spend down until you have

$2,000, or let's get your kids in here and pay them as caregivers," you're missing the opportunity that the laws give you.

Congress wrote the laws to allow you to save significant assets in most cases, and that's what the elder law attorney does. They connect you to how the laws work so that you can get the benefits that congress created for you.

If you are going to meet with the lawyer, be prepared to pay a fee. Always ask what the fee for the first meeting will be. Be prepared to discuss some specific issues that are important to you or your family member. It is good to look for a lawyer with a few years' experience and local to your area. You can ask for references, so you can talk to others about the lawyer and his skills. Obtain a copy of their brochure so you can study it.

FROM THE EXPERT: *Marty Fogarty*

My experience has been that elder law attorneys are more affordable than typical estate-planning attorneys. The great thing about my practice is that I can help someone with $50 or someone with $5 million. There's no escaping those elder chapters of life. You can pass away, but for anyone who lives through those chapters of life, there is an elder transition going on.

CASE STUDY: LAW OFFICE OF WILLIAM J. BRISK

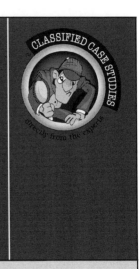

1340 Center Street Suite 205
Newton Centre, MA 02459
www.briskelderlaw.com
billbrisk@briskelderlaw.com
www.briskelderlaw.com
Phone (617) 244-4373
Fax (617) 630-1990

William J. Brisk—Certified Elder
Lawyer Attorney

Hopkins University in international and Latin American politics. He has taught elder law at Boston College School of Law. He has written three books on Massachusetts' elder law.

An increasing number of Medicaid appeals are necessary because applicants are being turned down more often. This is due to tougher qualification rules for Medicaid. When this happens they appeal the decision by having a fair hearing with Medicaid officials. It is important to have an elder lawyer or legal representation at the hearing to get some positive results. There are more denials of Medicaid funding these days than ever before. The five-year look-back period law makes it harder for seniors to give a gift to family and not have it counted or penalize them for Medicaid qualification.

All states now have estate recovery for Medicaid expenditures. Your home is an exempt asset when you apply for Medicaid. If you qualify for Medicaid and have long-term care , once you die, if you still own the house, the state can recover the medical expenses. If your spouse still lives there or you have a disabled child under 18 the estate will be exempt.

The Office of William J Brisk handles a variety of legal matter in elder law. They specialize in long-term care planning, estate planning, Medicaid eligibility, guardianship and litigation. William Brisk is a certified elder lawyer and belongs to National Academy of Elder Law Attorneys. He has a PhD from Johns

Long-term care insurance is a good idea for those who have assets to protect. Policies are frequently sold to people who have few resources and cannot afford the policy. You should not buy a policy if paying the premiums cuts into other basic living expenses. Policies have improved immensely and are a good source of money for long-term care at home. He advises purchasing a policy if you have the money to do so comfortably.

He believes most people do not need a trust. Some trusts are beneficial like a special needs trust for the disabled, testamentary trusts, and some tax related trusts. He believes many trusts are sold to those who do not need them. You must have enough assets to make them an effective planning tool.

The Law Office of William Brisk assists clients and families who face the physical and mental challenges of aging. With two decades of experience, they develop sound plans, implement them and when necessary litigate aggressively to protect the right of the elderly they represent.

What Is Certification and Is It Important?

The purpose of certification is to identify those individuals who have advanced knowledge, skills and experience in the area of elder law and/or retirement planning. The attorney must be certified to practice law in at least one state. He must have practiced law five years preceding the application and be a member in good standing with the bar where he or she is licensed. Attorneys must have spent at least 16 hours a week practicing elder law for three years preceding their application. In addition, they must have handled at least 60 elder law cases or matters in that time period.

The attorney must have continued or participated in educational seminars or courses in elder law for those three years. Attorneys must submit five references who are familiar with their competence and qualifications in elder law. Finally, the attorney must pass a full-day certification exam. The National Elder Law Foundations is the only organization certified by the ABA for Elder Law.

FROM THE EXPERT: *Marty Fogarty*

You don't need an elder law attorney who is "certified." You need someone who has been doing it for a long time, who can show you the math in about a half hour or 20 minutes, proving that you are in the equation to save and protect assets. Any elder lawyer worth his salt can do that. And if he can't do it, I don't care how many initials he has after his J.D., run away from him, and go talk to someone who can do that for you.

When you're talking about asset protection, the name of the game is certainty. It's, "If I pay you X number of dollars to create this trust, what is in it for me? What if I go to a nursing home tomorrow? What if I go in five years? Tell me what exactly the benefit is. Tell me that in dollars. Write it down." If they can't do that, run away from them. They're not the right guy for you. Because every elder lawyer should be able to do that for you.

Preparing to Meet an Elder Lawyer

Prepare for your meeting or you may waste your time and the attorney's. It can cost you money, because the lawyer will have to figure out why you are consulting him. It helps to have some idea of what you are seeking when consulting the elder lawyer.

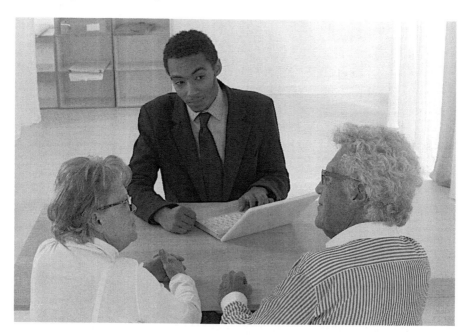

The attorneys will want to know who you are and why you are seeking help. Often, children contact a lawyer about helping their elderly parents. The lawyer will want to know the circumstance about the situation and if any other siblings are involved. He or she will want to know why the parent is not the one contacting him or her. If you have power of attorney, you will need to bring the document with you to prove that you have authority to seek help on your parent's behalf.

Sometimes a lawyer will send you a questionnaire in advance to gather information. Be sure to fill it out completely and send it there before your meeting, or bring it with you. Send copies to the lawyer's office or bring with you any copies of the documents requested in the forms you filled out.

Written documents are important to elder law. Some imperative documents might be copies of the power of attorney papers, wills, and trusts. If you applied for Medicaid, you may want to bring a copy of your paperwork to the meeting to go over. Spend some time thinking about what you might need for the meeting, and organize your paperwork.

Prepare a list of reasonable questions to ask the lawyer. Make sure you feel comfortable with the person before you commit to using them. Some questions you might ask are: what does the lawyer need to properly evaluate your case? Ask them to tell you how many similar cases they have handled. Can they tell some of the problems you will face in your case? How long will it take to handle your case and what is an estimate of the cost? Does the lawyer handle the case or give the case to an associate to handle?

CASE STUDY: THE KARP LAW FIRM

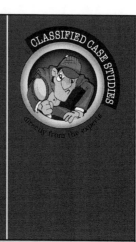

2875 PG Boulevard
Suite 100
Palm Beach Gardens, FL 33410
www.karplaw.com
Phone: (561) 625-1100
Fax: (561) 625-0060

Joseph S. Karp, Certified Elder Law
Attorney, Founder

The Karp Law Firm specializes in long-term planning for nursing home care, estate planning, wills, planning for special needs, disability planning, probate and trust administration for the elderly. Mr. Karp is qualified in the area of elder law. The Florida Bar and a member of the National Elder Law Foundation certify him as an elder law specialist. This is the only organization authorized by the American Bar Association. He was also a member and past president of American Association Trust, Estate and Elder Law Attorneys. His firm specializes in estate planning and asset protection for the elderly. They assist with Medicaid planning, too.

Mr. Karp recommends planning in advance. The sooner the better now that the look-back period is five years for Medicaid. He says Medicaid should really be a last resort. When talking about good trusts for the elderly he recommends the Irrevocable Income Only Trust. It gives the person control over their money or estate, provides protection from creditors, and allows for tax breaks. It reduces the risk of transferring assets directly to the children. Assets that can be transferred are homes, rental property, or liquid investments.

The solution to protect assets is to transfer assets to the irrevocable income only trust. The parents can name someone other than themselves as trustee and direct them to give money gifts to their children to use for their own long-term heath care. The individuals can make themselves trustees and keep control over the money giving themselves discretionary distributions from the trust. As trustees they would retain control over what is transferred into the trust giving them power and control of the assets. They have power to change the trustee if other than themselves and beneficiaries of the trust. They can receive income the trust generates but not the principal.

Mr. Karp says the irrevocable income only trust's benefit is that it avoids probate. It allows a step up basis or ability for the family to sell the trust tax-free after the owner's death. If you have the income you can keep enough to cover the nursing home for five years and the principal goes to the kid's when you pass away.

Mr. Karp strongly advises his elderly clients to purchase long-term health insurance as part of long term care planning. Talk to someone about the different long-term health insurance options don't wait until you are diagnosed with a serious medical disorder.

When purchasing a policy look at the cost of care in your community you income and assets. Try to make sure the policy has an inflation rider that covers the cost of living increases. If you purchase a policy keep it up especially as your grow older and may need the care. Many elderly people will drop a policy at 79 or 80 when they are most likely to need it. Look for a Partnership Plan that combines long term care insurance with Medicaid Extended Care. It allows you to protect some of your assets however in some cases income is countable. When making any plans for long-term health care Mr. Karp recommends consulting an experienced elder lawyer in your state.

FROM THE EXPERT: *Marty Fogarty*

If you're 50 years old and up, you're in the second half of your life, and you should be planning with an elder law attorney. There are two types of planning. There's pre-planning, and there's crisis planning. You want to do pre-planning because it's more affordable and you get more. Congress says that if you plan earlier, you get better options.

So, talk with an elder law attorney. Because when you're 50 and you're talking to your regular estate planning attorney, he's thinking about probates, he's thinking about estate tax, he's thinking about back-up trustees, etc. But your elder law attorney is thinking about all those things, and they're thinking about what else might go wrong in that elder transition. And your general estate-planning attorney doesn't know anything about that elder transition. That's going to be your number one threat in the decades of 60, 70, and 80. So you may as well plan with someone who specializes in dealing with that risk.

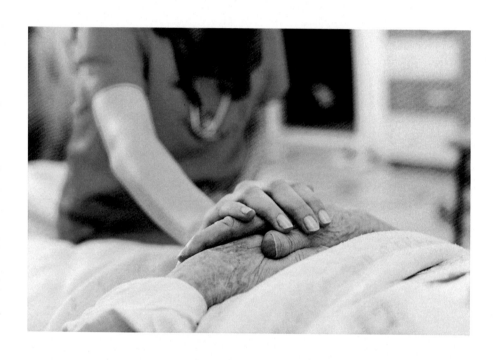

Chapter 9

Alzheimer's Disease & Medicaid

The Basics

It is estimated that by 2050, the number of people with Alzheimer's disease will reach up to 16 million. The epidemic threatens to bankrupt Medicare and Medicaid. According to the Alzheimer's Association, in 2016, the direct costs to American society of caring for patients with Alzheimer's and other dementias will total about $236 billion. Medicare and Medicaid cover about 68 percent of that total cost, totaling an estimated $160 billion.

When you break it down even further, we see that Medicaid alone is responsible for covering an estimated $43 billion caring for those with Alzheimer's and other dementias. This is an issue as the baby boom generation ages — the percentage of Americans with Alzheimer's is escalating quickly.

Medicaid is one of the few long-term care options available for this disease. Preventive care and hospital care are two required components of the program. The optional service is when states offer more than the required minimum, and often long-term care falls into this category. The optional groups include 80 to 90 percent of nursing home residents. When the economy is not doing well, these medical services are cut.

This can be devastating for those patients with Alzheimer disease and their families who require long-term care. The Alzheimer Association calls on Congress and the President to maintain Medicaid long-term care while expanding the home care options for patients like these. The group opposed the new plan to cut spending because it would affect this group and others like it that need assistance with long-term care.

The disease often takes years to progress. It causes a person to lose their ability to drive, work, and do normal activities that we take for granted. There is an increasing push for research to help slow the disease or find medicine to cure it. There have been federal hearings about the cost of long-term healthcare for victims of the disease. Research is not enough; families need to have long-term care options for this disease. It will not go away but will become a bigger problem as years go by.

FROM THE EXPERT: *Marty Fogarty*

The thing about Alzheimer's is that it's irreversible. It's generally a decline, and generally we have a little bit of time once we get that diagnosis.

I think the biggest challenge for Alzheimer patients is that there's a diagnosis for some sort of cognitive impairment, and then families have a choice. They can embrace it, go public with it, and come up with a strategy for how they're going to deal with it, or they can hide it, stuff it down, resist it, and not plan for it. Life gets worse when you do that. You have to embrace that diagnosis, you've got to be OK with the reality of what you've been diagnosed with, and you've got to make a plan going forward from there. And you can't do this alone. You need a support team for this.

Financial Planning

If you are employed, you should find out what coverage you have for long-term progressive diseases. If you do not have insurance, you should find out which ones have a high level of coverage for Alzheimer's disease. The Alzheimer's Association can help you with this question. If you are over 65, you can qualify for Medicare and can perhaps supplement it with another insurance through a private insurer; this insurance is often called Medigap. If your income is dangerously low, you may qualify for Medicaid; that is considered a government safety net.

It pays to investigate disability insurance and how much it would cost. You may eventually be unable to work, so this would provide you and your family with some income for the time when you can no longer work. You can check with your employer or a private insurance company to find out the cost of disability insurance.

For long-term care under Medicare, you must have stayed at least three days in a hospital. You must be admitted to a nursing home within 30 days of discharge from the hospital. You must enter the nursing facility with the same condition with which you were hospitalized. You must need daily skilled nursing care. The facility must be Medicare certified. Your physician must agree and design a care plan for you in the facility.

Often, patients with this disease need home care. Medicare covers home care if the patient is home bound. Care must be needed on a non-continuous basis. The care cannot exceed 35 hours a week or more than eight hours a day. If a person qualifies, they are entitled to a home health aide. Physical and speech therapy must be provided as needed.

If you have dreadfully low income, you may qualify for Medicaid. Some of the expenses covered are medications, care for hospital and doctors, medical supplies, health insurance premiums, and transportation for medical care. Medicaid coverage varies from state to state, and may cover home care services in some. When you apply within your individual state, you will find out what medical services are covered.

Long-term care insurance may be an option if you have time to shop for a policy and plan. The policies have improved and can assist you with home care and long-term assisted living or nursing home costs.

FROM THE EXPERT: *Marty Fogarty*

When the diagnosis occurs, my advice for those people is to get to an elder lawyer immediately. You need an advocate. Not just an elder lawyer. You need the elder lawyer to connect you to care managers, social workers, etc. So I've created a nonprofit organization called ElderSmart.net. You go there, and you can get the support, the connection, the guidance, and the assessment that says, "Given your circumstances, here's the order of priorities regarding what you should be doing."

There's no road map when it comes to Alzheimer's. If you had a heart attack because of a blocked artery, it's pretty easy. It's like going to Jiffy Lube. They say "Hey, we're just going to strip off these arteries, and we're going to replace them with these ones, and then we're all set to go." And then you're out. If you get an Alzheimer's or Parkinson's diagnosis, you don't know what to do. There are too many variables. Society, the medical community, and the health community have not been able to identify the path, and Elder Smart creates that path. The idea is to help educate and support families with a loved one in an elderly transition situation so that they can honor, support, and understand each other and that family member.

Type of Long-Term Care of Alzheimer's Patients

In Arizona, the Medicare Advantage Special Needs Plan designed a program for patients with Alzheimer's disease and chronic dementia. This health plan will offer residents special prescription drug coverage and care managers who specialize in memory disorders; the plan is managed through the health provider Evercare. The plan is designed to meet special needs of families dealing with the Alzheimer's disease. This includes a care manager who addresses financial planning, support groups for caregivers, emergency respite care, medications, and other needed therapies. Members will meet with Alzheimer specialists and have access to the latest drug treatments and methods available. This is a unique program developed for this disease.

Long-term care for Alzheimer's disease may mean getting help at home or moving your family member to an assisted living center or nursing home; there are more options available than ever before. If you decide to keep your family member living at home, some of these services may be helpful.

Community organizations or residential faculties often offer respite care. Sometimes, families, friends and neighbors can help. Adult day services programs are designed for Alzheimer's patients covered under Medicare or Medicaid and private insurance. They have qualified medical staff providing programs and meals for patients. Always make sure they have qualified staff to handle this illness. Some programs may not be qualified but take patients when they should not. Home health services involve personal care with bathing, dressing, cooking and other needed services.

Residential care options for Alzheimer's patients might include retirement housing for some patients in the early stages that can live alone, but not manage a house. It involves as small apartment, often with a kitchen or meals services. Sometimes, medical help is available from staff or a monitoring system. Often, social activities and other services are provided.

Assisted living centers are designed to provide some care but patients must not need 24-hour nursing level care. There are more centers designed for Alzheimer's disease, but make sure the proper medical staff is on-hand before you sign your family member up to live in an assisted living center. Specialized dementia care facilities may benefit those who need memory care assistance. It offers qualified medical personnel and special activities and programs for those with this illness. Nursing homes for those who need 24-hour care and skilled nursing are always available. Some facilities have special units for Alzheimer's disease with activities and programs designed for the individuals in it. For more information, contact your local Alzheimer's Association, which are excellent sources of information about programs and services in your local region.

FROM THE EXPERT: *Marty Fogarty*

I have created a nonprofit organization that supports people on this. Personally, I've lost two aunts and my dad to Alzheimer's. I've probably had hundreds of clients pass away over the last 16 years as well. So, I really feel like I have an insight to this that's unique. Because I'm the lawyer, I talk to these people beforehand, and then they pass away. I'm along for the ride, for the journey, to some degree. With my dad, I was the son with an out-of-state dad going through this, so I feel like I know something about what these kids are going through.

My dad chose not to share the information, which is very common, and it is still the basic way we're going to handle it in this country. And my experience is that choosing to hide it is choosing to resist and "fight it." I'm not saying we should just roll over and let it crush us, but I'm saying that if we allow it to be what it is, and not put negative pressure on it, I think that the transition can be better, less heart-wrenching, and less agonizing for the family. It's still a brutal disease. Society has not figured out how to deal with it, it's just absolutely heartbreaking to see your loved one go through it.

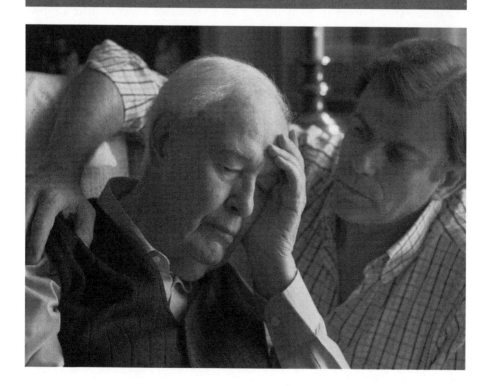

Where to Contact the Agency in Your State

Alabama

Alabama Medicaid Agency
501 Dexter Avenue
Montgomery, AL 36103-5624

Phone: 334-242-5000
Eligibility contact: 800-362-1504
Website: **www.medicaid.alabama.gov**

Alaska

State of Alaska Health and Social
   Services
Medicaid Program
P.O. Box 110640
Juneau, AK 99811-0640

Phone: 907-465-3347
Fax: 465-5154
Website: **health.hss.state.ak.us/dpa/
   programs/medicaid**

Arizona

Arizona Healthcare Cost Containment
   System
801 East Jefferson Street
Phoenix, AZ 85034

Phone: 602-417-4000
In-state outside Maricopa County:
   800-654-8713
Website: **www.azahcccs.gov**

Arkansas

Arkansas Medicaid
Department of Medical Services
Department of Human Services
P. O. Box 1437, Slot S401
Little Rock, AR 72203-1437

Phone: 682-8501 local and out-of-state
Toll Free: 1-800-482-5431
TDD: 501-682-6789
Fax: 501-682-1197
Website: **www.medicaid.state.ar.us**

California

California.gov Department of Health
Medi-Cal California Medicaid
   Program

Provider Enrollment Division
P.O. Box 997413
MS Code 4704
Sacramento, CA 95899-7413

Phone: 916-323-1945
Automated phone center:
    800-786-4346
Website: **www.medi-cal.ca.gov/
    sitemap.asp**

Colorado
Department of Healthcare Policy and
    Financing
1570 Grant Street
Denver, CO 80203

Phone: 303-866-3513
Toll-free: 800-221-3943
Website: **www.chcpf.state.co.us/
    default.asp**

Connecticut
State of Connecticut
Department of Social Services
25 Sigourney Street
Hartford, CT 06106-5033

Phone: 800-842-1508
Website: **www.ct.gov/dss/cwp/view
    .asp?a=2353&q=305218**

Delaware
Delaware Health and Social Services
Division of Medicaid & Medical
    Assistance

Harry Hill, Director
Pam Tyranski, Deputy Director
1901 N. Du Pont Highway, Lewis Bldg.
New Castle, DE 19720

Phone: 302-255-9500
Fax: 302-255-4454
Website: **www.dhss.delaware.gov/
    dhss/dmma/index.html**

District of Columbia
Department of Health
Government of the District of
    Columbia
825 North Capitol Street NE
Washington, DC 20002

Phone: 202-671-5000
Fax: 202-442-4788
Website: **http://doh.dc.gov**

Florida
Florida Agency For Healthcare
    Administration
2727 Mahan Drive
Tallahassee, FL 32308

Phone: 888-419-3456
Website: **www.fdhc.state.fl.us/
    Medicaid/index.shtml**

Georgia
Georgia Department of Community
    Health
2 Peachtree Street
Atlanta, GA 30303

Office of Rural Health Services
502 Seventh Street South
Cordele, GA 31015-1443

Phone: 404-298-1228
Toll-free: 800-766-4456
Website: **dch.georgia.gov/02/dch/
home/0,2467,31446711,00.html**

Hawaii

State of Hawaii
Department of Human Services
Med-Quest Division
801 Dillingham Boulevard, 3rd Floor
Honolulu, HI 96817-4582

Phone: 808-587-3521 or
808-587-3540
Fax: 808-587-3543
Website: **www.med-quest.us**

Idaho

Idaho Department of Health and
Welfare
Regional Medicaid Services
(including Personal Care Services)
1120 Ironwood Drive, Suite 102
Coeur d'Alene, ID 83814

Phone: 208-769-1567
Fax: 208-666-6856
Website: **healthandwelfare.idaho
.gov/Medical/Medicaid/tabid/
123/Default.aspx**

Illinois

Illinois Department of Healthcare and
Family Services
Department of Human Services
100 South Grand Avenue East
Springfield, IL 62762

Phone: 217-557-1601
Website: **www.dhs.state.il.us/page
.aspx?item=30359**

Indiana

Indiana Health Coverage Program
EDS Provider Enrollment and Waiver
P.O. Box 7263
Indianapolis, IN 46207-7263

Claims — EDS Customer Assistance:
317-655-3240 or 800-577-1278
Member Services: 877-633-7353,
Option 1
PA: 800-269-5720
Website: **www.indianamedicaid.com/
ihcp/index.asp**

Iowa

Iowa Department of Human Services
409 North 4th Street
Burlington, IO 52601

Phone: 515-256-4606
Toll Free: 800-338-8366
Fax: 319-754-4628
Website: **dhs.iowa.gov/ime/members**

Kansas

Kansas Health Policy Authority
Suite 900-N
Landon State Office Building
900 SW Jackson Street
Topeka, KS 66612

Phone: 785-296-3981
Website: **www.kmap-state-ks.us**

Kentucky

Kentucky Cabinet for Health and
    Family Services
Office of the Secretary
275 East Main Street
Frankfort, KY 40621

Phone: 502-564-5497
Fax: 502-564-9523
Website: **chfs.ky.gov/dms**

Louisiana

Lousiana Department of Health
628 N. 4th Street
P. O. Box 629
Baton Rouge, LA 70821-9030

Phone: 225-342-5774
Fax: 225-342-3893
Website: **ldh.louisiana.gov/index
    .cfm/subhome/1**

Maine

Maine Department of Health and
    Human Services
Office of MaineCare Services

442 Civic Center Drive
11 State House Station
Augusta, ME 04333-0011

Phone: 207-287-9202
Member Services: 800-977-6740
Website: **www.maine.gov/dhhs/oms**

Maryland

Maryland Department of Health and
    Mental Hygiene
201 West Preston Street
Baltimore, MD 21202

Phone: 877-463-3464
Website: **www.dhmh.state.md.us**

Massachusetts

Health and Human Services
Office of Medicaid
One Ashburton Place
11th Floor
Boston, MA 02108

Phone: 617-573-1770
Website: **www.mass.
    gov/?pageID=eohhs2homepage
    &L=1&L0=Home&sid=Eeohhs2**

Minnesota

Minnesota Department of Human
    Services
Aging and Adult Services
P.O. Box 64976
St. Paul, MN 55164-0976

Phone: 651-431-2670
Fax: 651-431-7453
Website: **mn.gov/dhs/people-we
-serve/seniors/health-care/health
-care-programs/programs-and
-services/medical-assistance.jsp**

Mississippi

Division of Medicaid
Sillers Building
550 High Street
Suite 1000
Jackson, MS 39201-1399

Phone: 601-359-6050
Website: **medicaid.ms.gov**

Missouri

Missouri Department of Social
  Services
221 West High Street
P.O. Box 1527
Jefferson City, MO 65102-1527

Phone: 855-373-4636
Aging Information Referral Line:
  800-235-5503
Website: **www.dss.mo.gov/fsd/
  msmed.htm**

Montana

Montana Department of Health and
  Human Services
Provider Relations Unit
P.O. Box 4936
Helena, MT 59604

Phone: 1-888-706-1535
Helena: 406-442-1837
Aging Services Network:
  800-551-3191
Fax: 406-442-4402
Website: **dphhs.mt.gov/Montana
  HealthcarePrograms/Member
  Services**

Nebraska

Nebraska Department of Health and
  Human Services
301 Centennial Mall South
Lincoln, NE 68509

Phone: 402-471-3121
Website: **dhhs.ne.gov/medicaid/
  Pages/medicaid_index.aspx**

Nevada

Nevada Department of Health and
  Human Services
Carson City
1100 East William Street
Suite 101
Carson City, NV 89701

Phone: 775-684-3676
Website: **www.medicaid.nv.gov**

New Jersey

Department of Human Services
Division of Medical Assistance &
  Health Services
Quakerbridge Plaza
P.O. Box 712
Trenton, N.J 08625-0712

Phone: 800-356-1561

Website: **www.state.nj.us
   /humanservices/index.shtml**

New Mexico

N.M. Human Services Department
2009 S. Pacheco Pollon Plaza
Sante Fe, NM 87504

Phone: 888-997-2583
Website: **www.hsd.state.nm.us**

New York

Department of Health
Corning Tower
Empire State Plaza
Albany, NY 12237

Phone: 718-557-1399 or
   877-472-8411
Website: **www.health.state.ny.us/
   health_care/medicaid/index.htm**

North Carolina

North Carolina Division of Medical
   Assistance
Division of Medical Assistance
1985 Umstead Drive
Raleigh, NC 27626

Phone: 919-855-4100
DHHS Customer Service:
   800-662-7030
Website: **dma.ncdhhs.gov/medicaid**

North Dakota

Department of Human Services
600 East Boulevard Avenue, Dept. 325
Bismarck, ND 58505-0250

Phone: 701-328-2310
Toll-free: 800-472-2622
Fax: 701-328-2359
Website: **www.nd.gov/dhs/about/
   contact.html**

Ohio

Ohio Department of Job and Family
   Services
30 East Broad Street, 32nd Floor
Columbus, OH 43215-3414

Phone: 800-324-8680
Website: **medicaid.ohio.gov**

Oklahoma

Oklahoma Healthcare Authority
4545 N. Lincoln Blvd, Ste. 124
Oklahoma City, OK 73105

Phone: 405-522-7300
Website: **okhca.org**

Oregon

Department of Human Services
Health Systems Division
500 Summer Street NE
Portland, OR 97301-1079

Phone: 503-945-5772
Website: **www.oregon.gov/oha/
   healthplan/pages/stateplan.aspx**

Pennsylvania

Pennslyvania Department of Human
  Services
Office of Medical Assistance Programs
P. O. Box 2675
Harrisburg, PA 17105-2675

Phone: 866-550-4355
Long-term Care Helpline:
  800-753-8827
Website: **www.dhs.pa.gov/citizens/
  healthcaremedicalassistance**

Puerto Rico

Medicaid Office of Puerto Rico and
  Virgin Islands
GPO Box 70184
San Juan, PR 00936

Phone: 212-616-2400
Website: **www.medicaid.pr.gov/
  Elegibilidad/SoyElegible.aspx**
  (Spanish)

Rhode Island

Rhode Island Department of Human
  Services
600 New London Avenue
Cranston, RI 02920

Phone: 855-840-4774
Website: **healthyrhode.ri.gov**

South Carolina

South Carolina Department of Health
  and Human Services

P.O. Box 8206
Columbia, SC 29202-8206

Phone: 888-549-0820
Website: **www.scdhhs.gov**

South Dakota

South Dakota Department of Social
  Services
700 Governors Drive
Pierre, SD 57501

Phone: 605-773-3165
Website: **dss.sd.gov**

Tennessee

Bureau of TennCare
310 Great Circle Road
Nashville, TN 37243

Phone: 800-342-3145
Website: **www.tn.gov/tenncare**

Texas

Texas Health and Human Services
Brown-Heatly Building
4900 N. Lamar Blvd.
Austin, TX 78751-2316

Phone: 512-424-6500
Department of Disability and Aging
  Services: 512-438-3011
Medicaid Client Hotline:
  800-252-8263
Website: **hhs.texas.gov/services/
  health/medicaid-and-chip**

Utah

Utah Department of Health
Utah Medicaid Program
Cannon Health Building
(Main Utah Department of Health
 office building)
288 North 1460 West
Salt Lake City, UT

Phone: 800-662-9651
Website: **health.utah.gov**

Vermont

Vermont Department of Children and
 Families
Economic Services Division
103 South Main Street
Waterbury, VT 05676-1201

Phone: 888-693-3211
Website: **www.vtmedicaid.com**

Virginia

Virginia Department of Medical
 Assistance Services
600 East Broad Street
Richmond, VA 23219

Phone: 804-786-7933
Website: **www.dmas.virginia.gov**

Washington

Washington State Department of
 Social and Health Services
DSHS Constituent Services
P.O. Box 45130
Olympia, WA 98504-5130

Phone: 800-562-3022
Website: **www.hca.wa.gov/free
 -or-low-cost-health-care/
 apple-health-medicaid-coverage**

West Virginia

West Virginia Health and Human
 Resources
Bureau for Medical Services
Office of Medicaid Managed Care
Room 251
350 Capitol Street
Charleston, WV 25301-3708

Phone: 304-558-6006
Website: **www.wvdhhr.org/bms**

Wisconsin

Wisconsin Department of Health
 Services
1 W. Wilson Street
Madison, WI 53703

Phone: 608-266-1865
Medicaid Hotline: 800-362-3002
Website: **www.dhs.wisconsin.gov/
 medicaid/index.htm**

Wyoming

Wyoming Department of Health
Qwest Building
6101 Yellowstone Road, Ste. 210
Cheyenne, WY 82002

Phone: 307-772-8401
Website: **wyequalitycare.acs-inc.com**

Appendix B

Medicaid News From
State to State

State and federal laws are constantly shifting and amending and changing—so, while we have done our best to provide you with Medicaid news from state to state, it's in your best interest to seek out professional help and advice through a company such as Elder Care Resource Planning (**www.eldercareresourceplanning.org**). Nevertheless, this section of this book will give you a brief overview of what each state has recently changes in terms of their Medicaid laws.

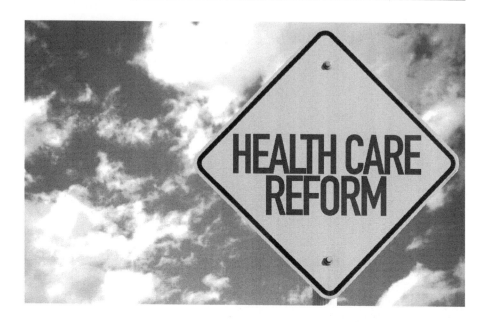

The expansion of Medicaid eligibility to anyone living below 138 percent of the federal poverty level was one of the cornerstones of the Affordable Care Act. However, the Supreme Court's 2012 decision to uphold the ACA stipulated that states had the right to choose whether or not to expand Medicaid, and that the government could not withdraw existing Medicaid funds if a state opted out of expansion. Those already eligible for or covered by Medicaid would not be affected by their state's choice to opt out; however, those whose income was too high for Medicaid but too low to purchase their own insurance would not be covered.

As of July 2016, 32 states have adopted Medicaid expansion and extended Medicaid coverage to low-income adults. The following 19 have chosen not to expand Medicaid:

- Alabama

  Alabama chose not to expand Medicaid coverage to low-income adults. Children, pregnant women at 141 percent of FPL, and parents or caretakers at 13 percent of the FPL are eligible. The federally-facilitated marketplace (FFM) also offers coverage in Alabama.

- Florida

  Florida chose not to expand Medicaid coverage to low-income adults. Children, pregnant women at 191 percent of FPL are eligible, as are parents or caretakers at 29 percent of the FPL. The FFM also offers coverage in Florida.

- Georgia

  Georgia chose not to expand Medicaid coverage to low-income adults. Children, pregnant women at 220 percent of FPL, and parents or caretakers at 34 percent of the FPL are eligible. The FFM also offers coverage in Georgia.

- Idaho

  Idaho chose not to expand Medicaid coverage to low-income adults. Children, pregnant women at 133 percent of FPL, and parents or caretakers at 24 percent of the FPL are eligible. A state-based marketplace also offers coverage in Idaho.

- Kansas

  Kansas chose not to expand Medicaid coverage to low-income adults. Children, pregnant women at 166 percent of FPL, and parents or caretakers at 33 percent of the FPL are eligible. The FFM also offers coverage through a partnership model in which Kansas takes over some of the aspects of health plan management.

- Maine

  Maine chose not to expand Medicaid coverage to low-income adults. Children, pregnant women at 209 percent of FPL, and parents or caretakers at 100 percent of the FPL are eligible. Insurance is also available through a partnership between the FFM and the state, which assume some plan management aspects.

- Mississippi

  Mississippi chose not to expand Medicaid coverage to low-income adults. Children, pregnant women at 194 percent of

FPL, and parents or caretakers at 23 percent of the FPL
are eligible. Insurance is also available through the FFM
and a state-based Small Business Health Options (SHOP)
marketplace, where small business owners and their employees
may shop for coverage.

- Missouri

  Missouri chose not to expand Medicaid coverage to low-
  income adults. Children, pregnant women at 196 percent of
  FPL, and parents or caretakers at 18 percent of the FPL are
  eligible. The FFM also offers coverage.

- Nebraska

  Nebraska chose not to expand Medicaid coverage to low-
  income adults. Children, pregnant women at 194 percent of
  FPL, and parents or caretakers at 58 percent of the FPL are
  eligible. The FFM also offers coverage through a partnership
  model in which Nebraska takes over some of the aspects of
  health plan management.

- North Carolina

  North Carolina chose not to expand Medicaid coverage to low-
  income adults. Children, pregnant women at 196 percent of
  FPL, and parents or caretakers at 44 percent of the FPL are
  eligible. The FFM also offers coverage.

- Oklahoma

  Oklahoma chose not to expand Medicaid coverage to low-
  income adults. Children, pregnant women at 133 percent of
  FPL, and parents or caretakers at 41 percent of the FPL are
  eligible. The FFM also offers coverage.

- South Carolina

  South Carolina chose not to expand Medicaid coverage to low-
  income adults. Children, pregnant women at 194 percent of

FPL, and parents or caretakers at 62 percent of the FPL are eligible. The FFM also offers coverage in South Carolina.

- South Dakota

  South Dakota chose not to expand Medicaid coverage to low-income adults. Children, pregnant women at 133 percent of FPL, and parents or caretakers at 57 percent of the FPL are eligible. The FFM also offers coverage through a partnership model in which South Dakota takes over some of the aspects of health plan management.

- Tennessee

  Tennessee chose not to expand Medicaid coverage to low-income adults. Children, pregnant women at 195 percent of FPL, and parents or caretakers at 103 percent of the FPL are eligible. The FFM also offers coverage in Tennessee.

- Texas

  Texas chose not to expand Medicaid coverage to low-income adults. Children, pregnant women at 198 percent of FPL, and parents or caretakers at 15 percent of the FPL are eligible. The FFM also offers coverage.

- Utah

  Utah chose not to expand Medicaid coverage to low-income adults. Children, pregnant women at 139 percent of FPL, and parents or caretakers at 44 percent of the FPL are eligible. In addition to FFM coverage options, Utah also uses a Small Business Health Options marketplace, where small business owners and their employees can shop for coverage.

- Virginia

  Virginia chose not to expand Medicaid coverage to low-income adults. Children, pregnant women at 1443 percent of FPL, and parents or caretakers at 49 percent of the FPL are eligible. The FFM also offers coverage through a partnership model in which Virginia takes over some of the aspects of health plan management.

- Wisconsin

  Wisconsin chose not to expand Medicaid coverage to low-income adults. Children, pregnant women at 301 percent of FPL, and parents or caretakers at 95 percent of the FPL are eligible. The FFM also offers coverage.

- Wyoming

  Wyoming chose not to expand Medicaid coverage to low-income adults. Children, pregnant women at 154 percent of FPL, and parents or caretakers at 55 percent of the FPL are eligible. The FFM also offers coverage.

A report from the State Health Reform Assistance Network, which is a Robert Wood Johnson Foundation program, found that states that chose to expand Medicaid saved money and generated revenue, which allowed them to either pay for the cost of expansion, or finance other state projects. Individuals who used to access state-funded services for the uninsured are now covered by Medicaid, and the vast majority of Medicaid dollars are paid for by the federal government. States can count on continued support from the government. Additionally, Medicaid expansion has created jobs in the healthcare and social service sectors.

States who chose to expand had flexibility in doing so, and a number of states have designed their own expansion programs. Arkansas, Iowa, Indiana, Michigan, Montana, and New Hampshire all have made additional changes using Section 1115 waivers. These waivers allow states to write in their own policies, including policies that address premiums, health savings accounts (HSAs), the ability to use Medicaid funds to buy private insurance, and incentivizing healthy habits. If you live in a state that has expanded Medicaid through an 1115 waiver, explore your state's Medicaid information webpage to learn about their alternative policies.

To see up-to-date, state-by-state information regarding changes to Medicaid, visit **www.medicaid.gov/state-resource-center/medicaid-state-plan-amendments/medicaid-state-plan-amendments.html**.

Bibliography

Alzheimer's Association. "Cost of Alzheimer's to Medicare and Medicaid." *Alz.org.* Alzheimer's Association, Mar. 2016. Web. 12 Sept. 2016.

Alexander J. Bove Jr., *The Medicaid Planning Handbook: A Guide to Protecting Your Assets From Catastrophic Costs* (Little Brown and Company), 1996.

Lita Epstein, MBA, *The Complete Idiot's Guide to Social Security and Medicare Second Edition*, (Alpha), 2006.

Diane Finch, "State Pilot Program Tests Alternatives to Nursing Homes," New Hampshire Public Radio, March 22, 2007.

Fogarty, Marty. "Medicaid and Elder Law." Telephone interview. 29 Sept. 2016.

Guerrero, Michael. "Medicaid and Elder Law." Telephone interview. 13 Sept. 2016.

Joan Harkins Conklin, *Medicare For The Clueless The Complete Guide to This Federal Program*, (Citadel Press), 2002.

K. Gabriel Heiser, Attorney, *How to Protect Your Family Assets from Devastating Nursing Home Costs MEDICAID SECRETS* (Phylius Press), 2007.

"Medicaid Expansion: Just the Facts." State Health Reform Assistance Network. April 2016. **http://statenetwork.org/wp-content/uploads/2016/03/State-Network-GMMB-Manatt-Medicaid-Expansion-Just-the-Facts-April-2016.pdf**.

Medicaid Program in Fifty States, **www.colorado2.com/medicaid/states.html**

National Conferences of State Legislatures; The Forum for American Ideas National Conference For State Legislatures.

National Elder Law Foundation Tuscon, Arizona, **www.nelf.org**

Piper Report Medicaid Medicare News 2008, **www.piperreport.com/about.html**

Sarah Baron. "10 Frequently Asked Questions About Medicaid Expansion." Center for American Progress. April 2013. **www.americanprogress.org/issues/healthcare/news/2013/04/02/58922/10-frequently-asked-questions-about-medicaid-expansion**.

Senior Journal on Medicaid New Tech Media, **www.seniorjournal.com/medicaid.htm**

"State Medicaid and CHIP Sponsors." Medicaid.gov. July 2016. Accessed October 2016. **www.medicaid.gov/medicaid-chip-program-information/by-state/by-state.html**.

"State Medicaid and CHIP Sponsors." Medicaid.gov. July 2016. **www.medicaid.gov/medicaid-chip-program-information/by-state/by-state.html**.

Glossary

Affordable Care Act (ACA): health care reform law in March 2010 (also known colloquially as "Obamacare"). This law has three goals: to make health insurance more affordable for all people, to expand the Medicaid program to cover all adults who fall under 138 percent of the poverty line, and to support new technological means of administering medical care to lower the costs of health insurance.

Affordable Coverage: job-based health plan covering only the employee that costs 9.66 percent or less of the employee's household income.

Benefits: health care items and services that are covered under the specific health insurance plan.

Broker: a person or business who can help an individual learn how to apply for coverage and enrollment in a Qualified Health Plan (QHP) through the Marketplace.

Caregivers: a person or organization that is responsible for the coordination of treatment across several health care providers for the patient who is seeking medical attention.

Centers for Medicare & Medicaid Services (CMS): federal agency that runs Medicare, Medicaid, and Children's Health Insurance programs.

Children's Health Insurance Program (CHIP): Insurance program that provides low-cost health coverage to children whose parents earn too much to qualify for Medicaid.

Claim: a request for payment, either by you or the health care provider, that is submitted to the health insurance company in order to receive coverage.

COBRA: a federal law that may allow you to temporarily keep your health insurance after you have been laid off or fired, you lose coverage as a dependent of a covered employee, or another related qualifying event.

Coinsurance: the percent of costs you pay the health care provider after you have already paid your deductible. For example, 20 percent of the cost of a doctor's visit.

Community Spouse: the husband/wife of a Medicaid applicant.

Copayment: a fixed amount you pay at a health care facility every time, only after the deductible has been met.

Cost Sharing Reduction (CSR): a discount that lowers the amount you have to pay for copayments, coinsurance, and deductibles.

Deductible: the amount you pay the health care provider before your insurance plan starts to pay for your medical treatment.

Department of Health and Human Services (HHS): the federal agency that oversees CMS.

Dependent: a child or other person that a parent or relative may claim as a personal exemption on their tax return.

Elder Law: law in place to protect the elderly in regards to health care, legal issues, and long term care planning.

Eligibility Assessment: the Marketplace's way of verifying the personal information of an applicant in order to give them health insurance.

Exclusive Provider Organization (EPO) Plan: a managed care plan that is only covered under the umbrella of specific doctors, specialists, and facilities.

Exemption: people who qualify, either by economic hardships or family loss, do not have to pay the fee for their health insurance.

Family and Medical Leave Act (FMLA): a federal law that allows certain employees at least 12 weeks of protected leave from a job due to a serious illness or disability, to have or adopt a child, or to care for another family member.

Health Insurance Marketplace: a service that helps people shop for and find affordable health insurance that works for them and their family.

HIPAA Eligible Individual: the status you have after 18 months of continuous health insurance coverage.

Hospice Services: services that provide comfort and care to those in the last stages of a terminal illness and their families.

Insurance Co-Op: a non-profit company where the owners are also insured by the company.

Liens: any sort of public record.

Limited Cost Sharing Plan: a plan available to federally recognized tribes and Alaska Native Claims Settlement Act (ANCSA) shareholders regardless of income or eligibility.

Long-Term Care: services that include medical and non-medical means of care for those who are unable to perform basic activities of life, such as dressing and using the bathroom.

Look-back Period: any gifts, transfers, or assets made within the last five years of applying for insurance are subject to penalties.

Medicaid: insurance program that provides low-cost or free health coverage to low-income families.

Medicare: a federal health insurance program for those 65 and older and certain individuals with disabilities.

Miller Trusts: if an individual's income exceeds the lawful amount for Medicaid, the individual must create this trust.

Obamacare: See Affordable Care Act.

Original Medicare: a fee-for-service health plan with two parts: hospital insurance and medical insurance.

Out-of-Network Coinsurance: the percentage you pay for covered health care services to providers that are not within your network within your health insurance plan.

Out-of-Network Copayment: a fixed amount you pay for health care services from providers who do not have a contract with your health insurance.

Out-of-Pocket Estimate: an estimate you have to pay for your own health care or prescription drugs.

Out-of-pocket Maximum: the most you could pay for health care services in one plan year.

Pre-existing Condition Insurance Plan (PCIP): a program that will provide you with health care coverage if you have been uninsured for at least 6 months, you have a pre-existing condition, and you have been denied coverage by a private insurance company.

Primary Care: health services that provide a broad range of medical treatments to the individual.

Qualifying Life Event (QLE): a change in your life that can make you eligible for a Special Enrollment Period.

Retirement Benefit: a payment or series of payments that are available to you after you retire from work.

Rider: amendment to an insurance policy.

Risk Adjustment: the statistical process that takes into account the health status and health spending for enrollees when they are looking at health care outcomes and costs.

Snapshot Rule: the brief synopsis of the period in which there is Open Enrollment for individuals in need of health insurance and whether or not there will be an extension.

Social Security: a system that distributes financial benefits to retired or disabled people.

Special Enrollment Period (SEP): a time outside the Open Enrollment Period when you can sign up for health insurance.

Spend down: excess income. Individuals may qualify if they spend this amount on medical bills.

State Health Insurance Assistance Program (SHIP): a state program that gets funding from the federal government to provide free and local health insurance to those under Medicare.

Subsidized Coverage: health insurance available at reduced or no cost for people with incomes under a certain level.

Survivorship Deed: a legal document that establishes joint tenancy of property between two parties.

Trustee: an individual given control or powers of administration of a property with a legal obligation to administer it solely for the purposes specified.

Zero Cost Sharing Plan: a plan available to members of recognized tribes and Alaska Native Claims Settlement Act (ANCSA) shareholders whose income is between 100 and 300 percent of the federal poverty level and who qualify for premium tax credits.

Index

Adult day care: 9, 22, 24, 28, 52, 61, 136-139, 143

Adult day healthcare options: 9, 139

Advisers: 26

Affordable Care Act: 19, 33, 70, 188, 195, 197

Alabama: 21, 128, 179, 188

Alaska: 15, 179, 197, 198

Alternative healthcare: 9, 150, 151

Alzheimer's: 10, 18, 52, 133-136, 139-141, 149, 173, 174, 176, 177, 193

Annuities: 7, 9, 36, 43, 73, 77-83, 94, 98, 99, 114, 153, 160, 161

Application tips: 6, 42

Arizona: 20, 24, 66, 90, 176, 179, 194

Arkansas: 135, 179, 192

Asset protection: 7, 8, 13, 73, 74, 78, 86, 87, 89, 98, 99, 101, 163, 164, 168, 170, 203

Assets: 1, 2, 6, 9, 11, 13, 15, 16, 18, 30, 31, 34-45, 48, 49, 53, 54, 56, 58, 59, 62-66, 71-74, 78, 82-92, 94, 95, 97, 99, 101, 102, 104, 111, 112, 114, 115, 118, 119, 121, 144, 153-167, 170, 171, 193, 197

Assisted living center: 89, 120, 131-135, 176, 177

Beneficiary deed: 110

Burial: 49, 102, 155-157

California: 25, 27, 28, 109, 134, 135, 139, 141, 176, 179, 206

CDs: 7, 57, 73, 84, 96-98, 154

Certification: 9, 54, 141, 167, 204

Charitable Remainder Trust: 7, 93

Chronic illness: 15, 25, 54, 159

Colorado: 110, 128, 180

Community spouse: 9, 35, 36, 41, 58, 64, 83, 88, 90, 91, 155, 158, 159, 162, 196, 203

Connecticut: 15, 60, 129, 130, 180

Countable assets: 9, 48, 63, 65, 153, 156, 159

Creditors: 55, 74, 86, 89, 94, 107, 109, 111, 113, 116, 117, 170

Deathbed will: 8, 103
Deductible: 27, 28, 53, 54, 61, 196
Delaware: 180
Dementia: 18, 53, 61, 133, 135, 141, 149, 176, 177
Disability insurance: 175
DRA: 6, 55

Elder lawyers: 9, 57, 144, 163
Enhanced life estate deed: 109, 111
Equity-fixed annuities: 7, 78
Equity-indexed annuities: 7, 79, 80
Estate planning: 34, 87, 104, 163, 166, 170, 171
Excess income: 5, 13, 33, 48, 198
Excluded assets: 9, 154
Executor: 36, 37, 102

Financial planning: 10, 73, 174, 176
Fixed annuities: 7, 79
Florida: ii, 2, 13, 30, 70, 109, 113, 130, 134, 158, 159, 170, 180, 187, 189, 203, 204
Funeral: 36, 49, 102, 155, 156

Georgia: 112, 180, 181, 189
Gift splitting: 6, 59
Gift tax: 59, 60, 62, 72, 92, 93, 109-111, 116, 117, 120
Gift trusts: 6, 59
Gifting: 6, 55
Grantor irrevocable trust: 7, 89
Guaranteed bonds: 7, 73, 97, 98

Hardship waiver: 41, 42, 65
Hawaii: 181

Holographic will: 8, 101, 103
Home care programs: 9, 127
Home- and community-based services: 16, 21
Homestead: 111, 120

Idaho: 21, 181, 189
Illinois: 27, 181, 213
Immediate annuity: 7, 82
Indiana: 27, 113, 114, 181, 192
Iowa: 181, 192
Irrevocable life insurance trust: 7, 91, 93
Irrevocable trust: 7, 84, 85, 89, 156

Joint interest: 8, 119
Joint ownership: 8, 107, 108, 116, 120

Kansas: 182, 189
Kentucky: 25, 182

Lady bird deed: 8, 108, 109
Legislation: 2, 135, 139
Liens: 6, 40, 111, 112, 196
Life annuities: 7, 81
Life estate: 8, 108, 109, 111, 118, 119
Life insurance: 6, 7, 13, 57, 60, 73-76, 82, 91-93, 112, 114, 153, 156, 157, 162, 203
Limited family partnerships: 6, 71
Living will: 8, 103-106
Long-term care: 2, 6, 9-13, 16, 18, 21, 22, 28, 34, 35, 40, 46, 52, 54, 56, 58, 60, 61, 66, 74, 110,

112, 114, 120, 127, 130, 162-164, 166, 167, 173-176, 185, 197, 204

Look-back period: 6, 43, 55-60, 62, 63, 65, 84, 95, 114, 118, 160, 161, 166, 170, 197

Louisiana: 182

Maine: 182, 189

Married couple: 35, 41, 90, 108, 116, 140, 156

Maryland: 138, 182

Massachusetts: 38, 40, 57, 111, 112, 121, 144, 145, 156, 166, 182, 186

Meals on wheels: 26, 146

Med-Cal: 17, 135

Medi-Medi: 20, 27

Medicaid annuity: 7, 77, 83, 161

Medicaid fraud: 45-47

Medicare: 5, 12, 15, 18-20, 27-29, 43, 51, 66, 69, 70, 138, 139, 142, 163, 173-177, 193-195, 197, 198

Medicare Part A: 27, 29

Medicare Part B: 27, 28

Medication: 91, 131

Mental health: 25, 29, 58, 163

Michigan: 100, 111, 112, 192

Miller trust: 7, 33, 87

Minnesota: 25, 129, 145, 182

Mississippi: 183, 189

Missouri: 15, 47, 183, 190

Montana: 183, 192

National Elder Law Foundation: 164, 170, 194

Nebraska: 183, 190

Nevada: 183

New Hampshire: 127, 192, 193

New Jersey: 21, 67, 183, 187, 192, 197, 206

New Mexico: 130, 184

New York: 23, 26, 67, 46, 60, 114, 147, 184, 186-190, 198, 199, 205, 209, 204

Nonprofit organizations: 93, 94, 146, 147, 149

North Carolina: 56, 184, 190

North Dakota: 184

Ohio: 109, 130, 134, 136, 184, 205

Oklahoma: 135, 184, 190

Old age pension: 29

Oral will: 8, 103

Oregon: 114, 184, 187

Outright gifts: 7, 94

PACE: 19, 28, 29, 158

Paid caregivers: 6, 65

Penalty period: 6, 55, 56, 59, 63, 84

Pennsylvania: 112, 114, 185, 187

Power of attorney: 42, 52, 87, 104, 169

Prescription drugs: 20, 35, 46, 156, 197

Prescriptions: 29, 45, 46

Private annuity trust: 7, 83

Revocable living trust: 7, 88

Revocable trust: 34, 84, 85, 88, 89, 164

Rhode Island: 185

Self-probating will: 8, 103
Snapshot rule: 9, 159, 198
Social services: 29, 30, 129, 159, 179,
    180, 183, 185
South Carolina: 185, 190, 191
South Dakota: 185, 191
Special needs trust: 7, 90, 91, 167
Spend-down: 13, 43, 85
Surrogate designation: 8, 106
Survivorship deed: 8, 107, 198

Tenancy: 107, 108, 110, 111, 198
Tennessee: 135, 138, 139, 185, 191
Term certain annuities: 7, 82
Testamentary special needs trust: 7,
    90
Texas: 22, 70, 109, 134, 185, 191
Transfer gifts: 6, 63

Transfer tax: 6, 62
Transition: 84, 130, 165, 171, 176,
    178
Trustee: 7, 84, 86, 88, 89, 92-95,
    170, 198

Unavailable assets: 9, 157
Utah: 112, 113, 186, 191

Value of assets: 9, 94, 153
Vermont: 21, 108, 186
Virginia: 114, 134, 175, 186, 191,
    192

Washington: 22, 180, 186
West Virginia: 114, 186
Wisconsin: 186, 192, 203
Wyoming: 186, 192

About the Experts

Brandon Pike

Brandon Pike is a licensed Senior Service Representative in the state of Florida. He currently works for the largest privately owned health, life, and annuity senior-focused insurance agency in America. He specializes in the senior market with health insurance, life insurance, safe investments, and retirement planning.

Marty Fogarty

Marty Fogarty is the founder of The Heartland Law Firm, which helps families have greater clarity about the legal protections available to them. Fogarty's firm has a core specialty in helping families understand their planning options for wills, trusts, and estate plans.

Michael Guerrero

Michael Guerrero is the Senior Benefits Adviser at Elder Care Resource Planning. He works with families all across the country on planning for and applying to get their Medicaid benefits started for their elderly loved ones. He is often advising families on asset protection strategies, community spouse resource allowances, the range of care environments, and caregiver agreements and compensation.

Julie Northcutt

As an entrepreneur in digital media, Julie Northcutt launched Caregiverlist.com in 2008 to deliver the efficiencies of digital technology to senior care companies, professional senior caregivers, and families. Ms. Northcutt developed the concept for Caregiverlist.com while owning a senior home care agency, Chicagoland Caregivers, which she founded in 2001 and grew into a leading agency in the Chicagoland area, with inclusion on the Inc. 5000's list of fastest growing private companies. She sold the agency to LivHome, Inc. in 2007 in order to focus on developing Caregiverlist.com. Caregiverlist launched the first senior care industry web portal for nursing home costs and ratings.

William J. Brisk

William J. Brisk, Esq. has achieved virtually every honor available to an elder law attorney. He is a Certified Elder Law Attorney and one of fewer than 60 Fellows of the National Academy of Elder Law Attorneys (NAELA). He has co-authored three books on elder law and has written articles, case comments, and book reviews on virtually every aspect of elder law. Boston Magazine has recognized Bill as a "SuperLawyer" since 2005. Bill concentrates his practice on long-term care, Medicaid eligibility, guardianships, and litigation.

Joseph S. Karp

Mr. Karp is among the few Florida attorneys who have earned double certification in elder law. He has been practicing law in Florida since 1977 and has advised and assisted thousands of families. Mr. Karp's legal career began as an Assistant District Attorney in The Bronx, New York, and then as a Public Defender in Palm Beach County, Florida. He credits his work as a prosecuting attorney and defense attorney for helping him learn to listen to all sides of a story—a skill essential to effectively serving clients. Understanding family members' goals, hopes and fears is a prerequisite to developing an effective legal plan for any family. Mr. Karp is married and has two sons.